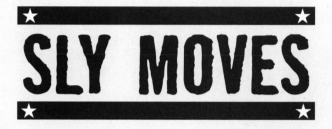

My Proven Program to Lose Weight, Build Strength, Gain Will Power, and Live Your Dream

SLY MOVES

BY SYLVESTER STALLONE

WITH DAVID HOCHMAN

This book is written as a source of information only. The information contained in this book should by no means be considered a substitute for the advice of a qualified medical professional, who should always be consulted before beginning any new diet, exercise, or other health program.

This book has been carefully researched, and all efforts have been made to ensure the accuracy of its information as of the date published. All of the procedures, poses, and postures should be carefully studied and clearly understood before attempting them at home. The author and the publisher expressly disclaim responsibility for any adverse effects, damages, or losses arising from the use or application of the information contained herein.

PHOTOGRAPH CREDITS
All photographs by Isabel Snyder except for those on the following pages:
Sylvester Stallone's Personal Collection: vi, 11, 13, 14, 18, 25. Hunter Martin: 3.
Tony Dizino: 8–9, 23, 184–185, 200. Courtesy of MGM CLIP+STILL: 21, 31.
Ken Regan: 22. Peter C. Borsari: 27. Courtesy of Ronald Reagan
Library: 35. George Pipasik: 36, 39. Roland Neveu: 41. Miramax Films: 43.
Todd Warshaw/Getty Images: 188. Denise Truscello/WireImage: 196.
Chris Haston/NBC Universal: 206. Dave Bjerke/NBC Universal, 208.

HarperCollins books may be purchased for educational, business, or sales promotional use. For information please write: Special Markets Department, HarperCollins Publishers, Inc., 10 East 53rd Street, New York, NY 10022.

FIRST EDITION

Designed by Timothy Shaner

Library of Congress Cataloging-in-Publication Data is available upon request.

ISBN 0-06-073787-5

05 06 07 08 09 ❖ 10 9 8 7 6 5 4 3 2 1

To all the people who changed my life—hopefully I can repay the favor. And to my family, who fill me with love—and drive me insane.

Thank you to Kevin King, Esther Newberg, Jeff Berg, Andrea Eastman, Kerry Pearse, Kathy Huck, Michelle Bega, Paul Bloch, and Megan Newman.

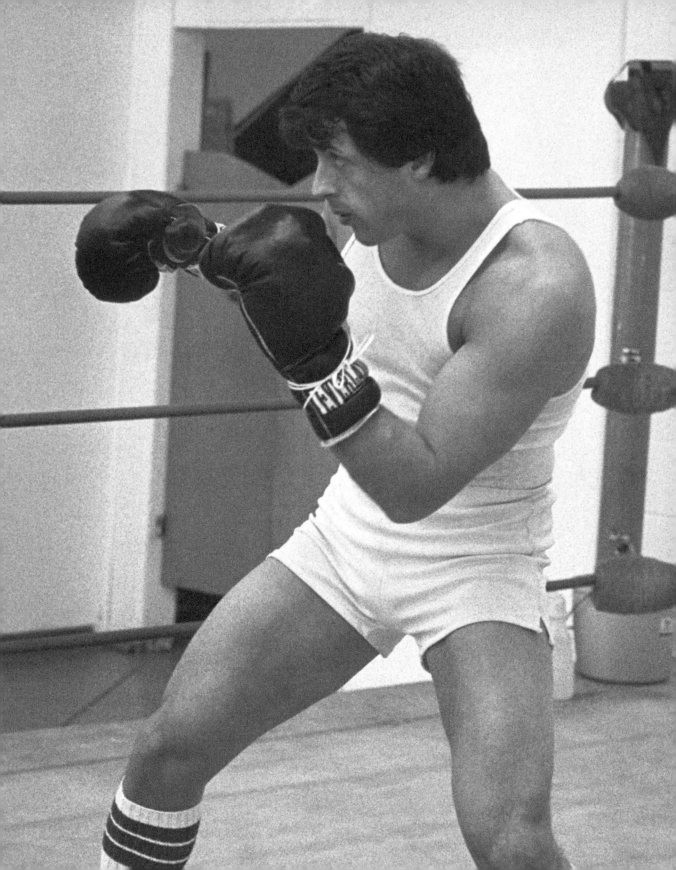

★ CONTENTS ★

★ CONTENTS ★

★ CONTENTS ★

INTRODUCTION:
THE ROCKY FACTOR

If there was any doubt about my place in pop culture, it was laid to rest the night I returned to Philadelphia in the fall of 2003 to dedicate the Eagles' new football stadium. Standing atop a tower over the north end zone, I looked out as 70,000 cheering fans told me exactly what was on their minds: "*Ro*-cky! *Ro*-cky! *Ro*-cky!"

I know that until the day I die I will be remembered for playing Rocky Balboa, the club fighter from South Philly who takes his million-to-one shot and goes the distance with the heavyweight champion of the world. No matter how many other movie roles I do (including Rambo) or projects I put my name on, the world will forever see me as that guy in the ugly gray sweats yelling "Yo, Adrian!" and bounding up the steps of the Philadelphia Museum of Art. When I was younger I fought it, now I embrace it.

Now I'm just thankful, because the Rocky philosophy is my ideal state, the immutable voice inside my head that says, "Never lose sight of what you want to be." So many people go through life with unrealized ambitions, reluctant to take the steps necessary to achieve true peace of mind, whatever that may be, because they have been overwhelmed by life's pressures. *Now it's time to grab life by the throat and not let go until you succeed.*

Through the years, as I changed my body for various roles and pushed myself toward more demanding physical challenges, I learned some extraordinary lessons about what works and what doesn't when it comes to diet, exercise, and mental attitude. That knowledge was hard earned, especially since there were no guidelines for my particular path in life. Nobody ever handed me a book on how to develop Rocky's abs, Rambo's back, or *Cliffhanger* legs. Or for gaining and losing 40 pounds, like I did for *Cop Land*. It was all a giant experiment and I was the guinea pig.

For a long time, I've wanted to put those valuable lessons on paper, to share what I've experienced in order to make it easier for others to transform themselves. The book in your hands is the end result of a lifetime of trial and error, of ups and downs on the way to building muscle, strength, power, energy, and clarity—without the pain and difficulty usually associated with dramatic change.

As you'll discover in Part I, a retrospective of how I've trained for various roles, I've tried practically every complicated diet and exercise regimen known to man only to realize the best ways to stay fit and feel great also happen to be the simplest. That's why my unique training plan goes back to basics. Parts II and III outline my programs for shaping up and eating smart. It's a stripped-down regimen that won't waste your time and absolutely *will* get you results. Part IV shows how you can put those simple techniques into action in every part of your life.

THE BODY OF A LIFETIME

When we're young, we think we can live forever. We sometimes pay attention to our bodies and sometimes don't. We eat well and exercise, or maybe we don't. Either way, most of us survive, since the body has a curious habit of taking care of itself. But by the time we reach 40, we need to make a choice: is it time to give in or are we ready to beat the clock?

Some people buy into the philosophy that you have a few good years before the next generation comes along and tells you to step aside. Don't believe that. The older we

RIGHT: Sly receives a warm welcome from Philadelphia Eagles fans in 2003.

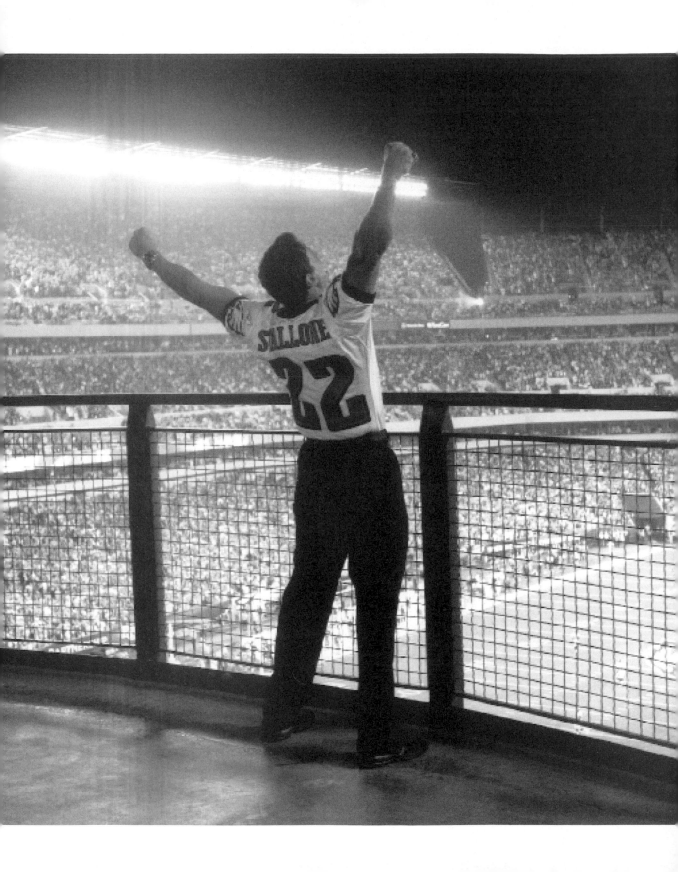

get, the smarter we get and the smarter we live. You can achieve extraordinary things into your fifties, seventies, and beyond if you really want to. It's that simple. All it takes is the desire to live better and the passion to feel more alive. It's that simple if you're prepared for it.

That's where health and fitness come in. The way you eat and exercise triggers an extraordinary amount of responses—physical, mental, and eventually spiritual. There is nothing that makes you feel more in touch with and proud of yourself in the long run as maintaining some sort of positive physical routine. Whether it's walking up and down three or four flights of stairs every day, saying no to unhealthy snacks, or lifting weights after a lifetime of inactivity, there's no better way to build an affirmative self-image. When you steadily build strength and treat your body right, when you do things you sometimes don't want to do, you ultimately triumph over the negative parts of yourself and arrive at a place where anything is possible. I say bring on the challenges.

If you're reading this and you're 25 or 30, you're probably saying, "What does he know?" I get that, because I felt the same way. I didn't want to take advice from anybody in my younger days. But believe me, unlike so many of the self-proclaimed fitness gurus out there, I've lived the life I preach. Health and fitness has gotten me through so many rough times and it's provided a will to take on every new challenge life has thrown at me. *Face it, the old cliché is true: no matter how rich or famous you are, without your health you've got nothing.*

IT'S OKAY TO BE BIG. JUST TRY TO STAY STRONG.

I don't have to tell you that obesity is a major problem in our society, but we've got to be realistic. As a country, as a planet, we won't be getting thinner anytime soon. Look around. Walk through any mall or airport in America. Supersizing is here to stay, and the sad part is the way food is processed and laced with chemicals, *which make you eat more.* Most people face an impossible task of keeping their weight down with the junk that's being passed off as food. But here's the encouraging news: our weight is not our health. I weigh 20 pounds more than I did when I made *Rocky*;

40 more than I did in *Rocky III*. But I've never felt better about my body and my health.

Some of the country's leading physiologists and nutritionists are discovering that exercising and eating smarter are more important to long-term well-being than losing weight. In the pages ahead, I will share with you some incredible research that shows how even overweight people can lower their risk of diseases such as diabetes and cancer by simply moving their bodies, even just a little. Three 10-minute walks a day can make a huge impact on how you look and feel. One study found that overweight people who exercise regularly outlive skinny people who don't—*by a ratio of 2 to 1.*

A big part of the equation is making a commitment to moving around on a regular basis, and that's all I ask of you. In the pages ahead, I'll share some of my favorite exercises and fitness strategies. Most of these routines have been around since the dawn of the dumbbell, and that's because they work exceptionally well no matter what your fitness level. There are classic, advanced, and women's workouts as well as a hard-core drill session for times when you need an extreme challenge. The best news is the program won't take more than three or four hours a week once you have it down—you'll love it, because you'll love the way you'll feel. If you're big, so be it. But maybe together, we can work out an enjoyable way to make you feel better than you did the day before.

I have a very active lifestyle. I go to the gym, I play with my kids, I chase my crazy dog around the yard. But I also eat everything I want *in moderation*. If I want ice cream, I'll have it. Pizza? Bring it on. It's purely a matter of finding a healthy balance, and I'll show you how that works. I firmly believe in *shaping up without giving up* the pleasures that make life worth living. I wouldn't give them up and wouldn't expect you to, either.

DIETS DON'T WORK!

The grapefruit diet, the cabbage soup diet, Atkins, South Beach, high-protein, low-protein, even high-altitude high-carb. I've tried them all and here's what I've discovered: *eventually every diet will let you down.*

According to the Federal Trade Commission, more than 95 percent of people who begin a weight-loss program each year regain their prediet weight—or put on more pounds. A 95 percent failure rate. That's almost as bad as the chances of becoming a very successful actor. Anyway, look around. If all those best-selling diet books are so effective, why can't most of us name five people who've lost a substantial amount of weight and *kept it off* for more than a year?

And yet we still diet, because most of us are shortsighted. When you go on a strict diet, you will lose weight quickly. Great, except it's mostly water and muscle, and that's *very bad*. Soon, the hunger pangs, the complicated preparation, the lack of flavor, and the miserable feeling drive you back to the same old habits and the same old waistline. And here's the kicker: unless you're exercising, the weight you gain back after a diet isn't that all-important muscle you lost, it's fat. You know that, yet out of frustration you go out desperately seeking a new "wonder" diet book. The *one* that promises the "miracle" formula that will change your life forever. No wonder weightloss products rake in more than a billion dollars a year and disappoint you time and again.

I gave up dieting years ago and I've never been more in control of my weight. Kicking the diet habit may be the smartest thing you can do to keep your body feeling great.

WHAT WOULD HERCULES DO?

If there were a law that said you had to eat one type of cuisine for the rest of your life, I bet the majority of us would choose Italian. And why not? It's great-tasting and, by the way, the healthiest. Human beings thrive on fresh fruits and seasonal vegetables, whole grains and legumes, olive oil as the primary fat source, fish, and small amounts of veal, lamb, and chicken. Rich in antioxidants, low in saturated fats and cholesterol, it's the diet that keeps on giving. And, yes, red wine is a good thing.

As you'll see when I show you my menu of meals in a typical week, I've been eating the same basic foods for 40 years. And while I've never been a gourmet, I've discovered a way to enjoy delicious foods without sacrificing my commitment to health. But it certainly helps that I give myself one day a week to eat *anything* without feeling guilty, and I'll show you how you can, too.

LIVE LIKE A CONTENDER

Feeling great is about taking control. It's about making a reasonable commitment. Only you can make the decision to get in shape, to start eating healthier and exercising more. In the final section of this book, I'll show you how to rise above years of limiting habits and set smart goals so you can overcome your biggest opponent in the fight to stay fit: yourself. The attitudes we develop toward food and exercise are so difficult to change, but even minor adjustments in how you treat your body can dramatically improve your long-term picture of health.

If you're looking to make changes in how you look and feel, if you want to increase your energy and improve your mood, there's no better time than right now. All those late-afternoon snack binges, the hours spent loafing on the couch, the unresolved New Year's resolutions . . . no problem. Here's your chance to clear the slate, to make changes in your body that will affect your mind in the most positive way for years to come. *Best of all, you can do it without turning your whole world upside down.*

★

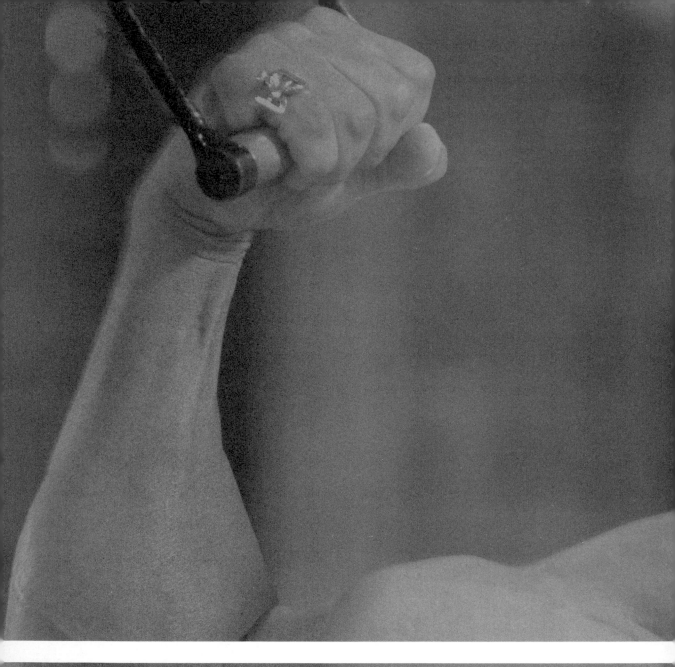

PART 1
SLY ON SLY

Winners get rid of their problems before their problems get rid of them.

THE MAKING OF A CONTENDER

Growing up in Silver Spring, Maryland, I'd spend my Saturday afternoons at the Silver Theatre, an old Arabian Nights–style movie palace, mesmerized by matinee idols like Commando Cody, Masked Marvel, and Sinbad the Sailor. Like the comic book characters I loved so much, these movie icons had powerful physiques that made them invincible, and as a 98-pound weakling, I couldn't get enough of their adventures. Still, none of them came close to making an impression like the mighty mortal they called Hercules.

I was 12 when I first saw Steve Reeves in *Hercules*, and I probably watched the movie 15 or 16 times that summer. My mind exploded! I saw a perfect physical specimen that was both heroic and human, and it was the first time in my life I started thinking about what I wanted to look like physically, how I wanted to develop in terms of proportions. So

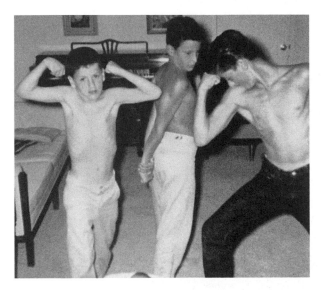

RIGHT: A young Sly (far left) poses with friends.

don't tell me films don't have a lasting impression on children. Sitting in that dark theater, being so enthralled by the images on that screen, is definitely the major reason I am here today.

★

My own life wasn't quite so heroic in those days. I was born in a clinic on Tenth Avenue and Forty-ninth Street in the Hell's Kitchen neighborhood of New York City in the boiling summer of 1946. A forceps accident at birth immobilized the motor nerves on the left side of my face, leaving me with a crooked mouth, a droopy eye, and this famous locution of mine.

As I got older, people teased me all the time and I became a chronic misbehaver. I wasn't a big kid or especially handsome. And with my speech problems and a name like Sylvester, life was becoming a cruel joke with no punch line in sight. I transferred from school to school because of behavioral problems; one teacher actually introduced me by saying, "Class, we have a new student today. His name is Sylvester, as in the cartoon." So for the rest of the year I got "Hey, Tweety Bird!" or "What's up, Poody Tat?" Nice, huh? A real confidence builder.

Back home, my father taught me how to be physically strong. Just watching him was a lesson in the power of kinetic energy. He didn't lift weights, but he'd constantly be moving rocks, cutting down trees, and pushing heavy machines around. There was nothing elegant about it, but the man was definitely in great shape. Country strong, they call it.

My mother, was also very physical, but she was a little more scientific about it. Her father was a district court judge who'd once roomed with Charles Atlas, the most famous bodybuilder ever. Mom started exercising with her father when she was very young, and she grew up hitting a punching bag and tossing around a medicine ball.

My mother is a chance taker, and one of the most unusual things she's ever done in her life was to open a women's gym in Washington, D.C., in 1954, when hardly anybody went to gyms. Especially not women.

When I was in sixth grade, I was so obsessed with the idea that I could become Superboy, I actually

RIGHT: Sly's mother, Jacqueline, at her gym, Barbella's.

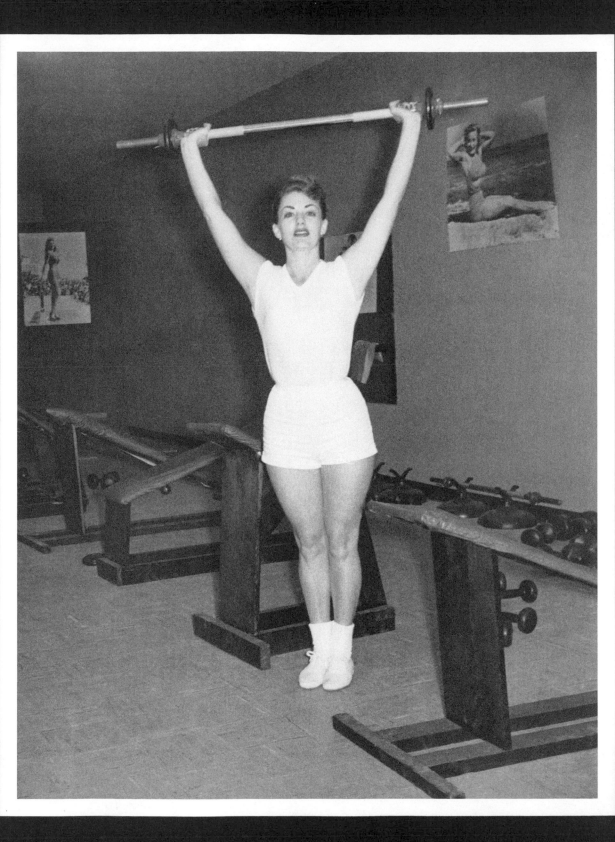

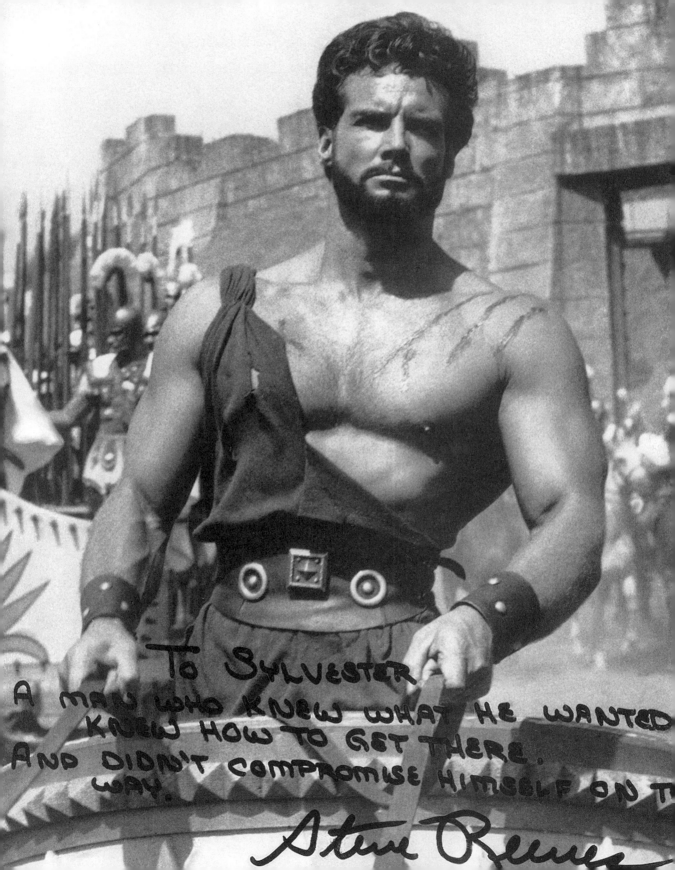

To Sylvester
A man who knew what he wanted
knew how to get there.
And didn't compromise himself on t
way.

Steve Reeves

tried to make it happen. I went out and bought some red dye and a wax crayon and painted a big *S* on a shirt. I found a barber's cape, dyed it red, and then slipped into a blue bathing suit. For days, I'd literally wear this crazy getup under my clothes. It was like I was telling myself that if I wished hard enough, the transformation would begin.

Unfortunately, I decided to share this top-secret information with my friend Jimmy. He promised and crossed his heart he'd never reveal this extraordinary information. Of course, he told the teacher. She brought me in front of the class. "Children, we have a special guest today, Superboy." She made me take my clothes off. As I stood in my baggy Speedo, everybody could see what a knock-kneed superhero pretender really looked like. After the laughter died down, I took my breadstick arms and pipe cleaner legs and blew out of there, my wrinkled cape flapping pathetically in the breeze.

But it didn't matter. I knew I'd found a superhero I could emulate in *Hercules*. It helped that Reeves was as impressive off screen as he was in the movie. The son of a farmer from Glasgow, Montana, he began body-building as a teenager and soon developed one of the most remarkable physiques around. After returning home from World War II, he racked up titles as Mr. America, Mr. World, and Mr. Universe before Hollywood made him the biggest action star of his day.

Later in my life, Reeves and I became friends. What I most admired about him was how modest he was. He was never a poser or a show-off. He wasn't one of those guys who announced to the world how fit he was. Steve wore oversized sweat suits. Best body in the world and he covered it up.

Reeves was the real deal, and his influence on my life was truly profound. Here at last was a way out of my awkward youth. If I wasn't happy with myself as I was, maybe—just maybe—I could sculpt myself into the person I wanted to be.

After one of those Saturday matinees, I decided to start building myself up, so I went to the town junkyard and just started lifting whatever I could find: a brake drum, half a fender, a steering column. I started tying rocks together with ropes. I'd do curls with cinder blocks strapped to a broom handle. My

LEFT: Sly's boyhood hero, Steve Reeves, playing the title role in Hercules.

A BIG THUMBS DOWN ON MOVIE FOOD

For many people, a movie just isn't a movie without movie food. When I was a kid, I couldn't set foot in a theater unless I had my two or three boxes of Jujyfruits and a bag of buttery popcorn. Washed down with a cold soft drink or two, it was a meal made in movie heaven—not exactly healthy, but a minor infraction compared with what it's morphed into.

The standard 1950s popcorn box had 3 cups of popcorn and about 174 calories. Today, popcorn comes in 21-cup tubs and pack as much as 1,700 calories. Soft drinks were 6.5 ounces back then. Now they're 16 or 32 ounces and have more than twice the calories. And there's a new generation of temptations for your viewing pleasure: cookie dough ice cream, sour cream and onion pretzels, nachos drowning in cheese sauce.

The psychology of movie food is fascinating. Once the lights go down, we think we have special dispensation to eat anything we want. It's almost like we're under a voodoo spell. Where else but at the movies do you kick back with a supersized box of Sno-Caps? Theater owners love it, of course, and I don't blame them. They make about 40 percent of their profits from concession sales. But next time you're in line for that giant box of blockbuster goodness, consider what's inside:

Reese's Pieces	8 oz	1,200 calories	60 g fat	138 g carbs
Skittles	6.75 oz	765 calories	9 g fat	166.5 g carbs
Twizzlers	6 oz	600 calories	4 g fat	136 g carbs
Goobers	3.5 oz	525 calories	35 g fat	55 g carbs
Raisinets	3.1 oz	380 calories	16 g fat	64 g carbs
Sno-Caps	3.1 oz	360 calories	16 g fat	60 g carbs
Milk Duds	3 oz	340 calories	12 g fat	56 g carbs
Junior Mints	3 oz	320 calories	5 g fat	68 g carbs

Popcorn

Remember that news flash a few years ago that said a tub of "buttered" movie popcorn has a whole day's worth of fat? While you may think theaters fixed the problem, think again. Most chains still use coconut oil or partially hydrogenated canola oil to pop their corn, according to the Center for Science in the Public Interest (CSPI), which first blew the whistle on movie popcorn in 1994. "A few theater chains switched to lower fat oils but many switched back and many others still use the 'bad' oils," says Jayne Hurley, CSPI's senior nutritionist. How bad is the problem? A large buttered popcorn has 1,500 to 1,700 calories and about 116 grams of fat. Sneaking in a bag of air-popped popcorn is a safer bet at only 30 calories per cup.

Incidentally, when the Silver Theatre of my youth was restored in 2003, new, wider seats had to be installed to make room for supersized cup holders, not to mention twenty-first-century backsides.

friends probably looked at me back then and thought, "Oh, this too shall pass."

Soon enough, I found this dungeon-like weight-lifting place called Iron City. We're talking *old* school. The town tough guys there would work out and smoke cigarettes at the same time. It was all iron bars, not a weight machine in sight. It was a hellhole to the passerby, but to me it was a godsend.

What I began realizing was that the body is nothing but an honest machine that will never cheat you. It gives back exactly what you give it, good or bad.

A MILLION-TO-ONE SHOT

Being an actor during my early days in New York was slow-going, so I spent most of my time doing odd jobs to pay the rent: cleaning lion cages at the zoo, slicing fish heads, whatever it took to get by. I auditioned for nearly every single casting agent in town but usually got rejected. The roles I did land were mainly the blink-and-miss-me type. I was the guy in

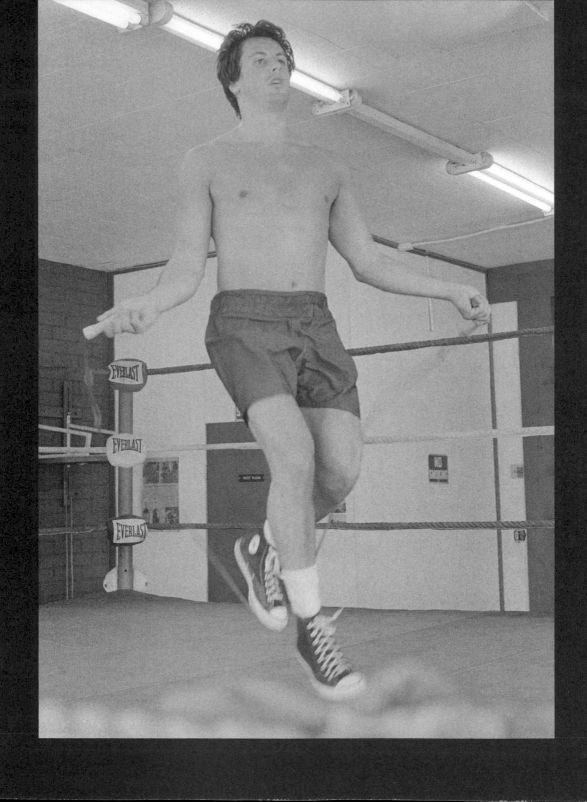

Bananas beating up Woody Allen on the subway, and the mugger who got mugged by Jack Lemmon in *The Prisoner of Second Avenue*.

I'd always known that physical appearance is very important in getting started in the movie business, and I also thought I could come up with different looks for different roles by experimenting with dieting and exercise. That really came into play in *The Lords of Flatbush* in the early seventies. I needed to morph into a hulking Brooklyn thug, so in the weeks before shooting, I went from 160 pounds to 200 pounds. It was probably the easiest weight-training regimen I ever had on a movie. Every day, I'd gorge on whatever was cheap and fattening. I didn't know better.

By the time I sat down to write the script for *Rocky* shortly after my twenty-ninth birthday, I had been exercising half my life, but in many ways I was just starting to learn about fitness. Up to that point, my workouts had been erratic and unorthodox, partly because I was flat broke and couldn't afford to get to a proper gym. I remember I had one of those crude 60-pound, turn-of-the-century dumbbells in my apartment. It was black and had *York, Pennsylvania* printed on the sides and a huge grip like one of those strongman weights you'd see in the circus. *That* was my health club.

Proper nutrition was an absolute mystery to me back then, too. All I knew was that fighters were strong, so I took the old-school approach and beefed up on fried chicken and potatoes, burgers and fries, spaghetti and baked ziti, whatever I thought would build muscle mass. If you recall, Rocky calls himself a "ham and egger," but he just as easily could have been an "ice cream–and–milkshaker," because that's what I was eating at the time—which made about as much sense scientifically as that cocktail of raw eggs I drank for breakfast in the movie. (Actually, that scene was a tribute to those early days in New York. I couldn't afford to eat out, so I kept eggs on my windowsill and learned to eat them raw.)

I was under the impression I was in great shape until I met Carl Weathers, the actor who played Apollo Creed. My body conditioning was basically average, and in some areas I was weak and out of shape. Looking back on some of the pictures from

LEFT: Early training for Rocky— *with a long way to go.*

that time is a cold slap in the face. How did I ever think I could pull off playing a veteran heavyweight with that body? My body was light-years behind. All I had was the desire and not much else. Sometimes it does help to be delusional. Anyway, I had originally wanted Ken Norton, a real heavyweight and former world champion, to play my opponent, but once Carl came into my office and threw a few jabs and hooks my way, I thought he might have a shot. When he took off his shirt, the deal was sealed. Standing next to him, I instantly became Kid Cannoli. Carl was chiseled. It was partly due to good genetics, but he also knew what he was doing, and I learned so much from him about physiology, diet, and exercising smarter. In the beginning, he knocked me around like a rag doll. The out-take footage of us boxing together is totally hilarious.

I've always said *Rocky* is semi-autobiographical. Having grown up in the streets, I knew a million down-and-outers. I knew what they ate, where they worked, how they thought. Most of all, I understood their broken dreams. I'm a guy who basically had to build himself from scratch. Fortunately, I'd always known how to work with what I had, and some-times that's all it took to achieve success: a little discipline and a little luck. And you know what? If you can relate to that, you're in the majority. That's the story of the planet.

At the same time, setbacks had always inspired me. In high school in Philadelphia, I went out for football and barely made the team. I was the least experienced player by far. But that made me say, "Let's see if I can become the strongest." The next year, after some of the best senior players moved on and after working on my game all summer, I became starting linebacker and captain.

It was that same spirit that carried me through the summer of 1975. I thought about all the people who fail to live up to their potential because they're too scared or intimidated or beaten down—I was thinking about myself, really—and I wrote the first *very* rough draft of *Rocky* in a three-and-a-half-day, coffee-drenched frenzy. It was a story I needed to get out.

RIGHT: Early rehearsals of Rocky going the distance.

I had $106 to my name and no

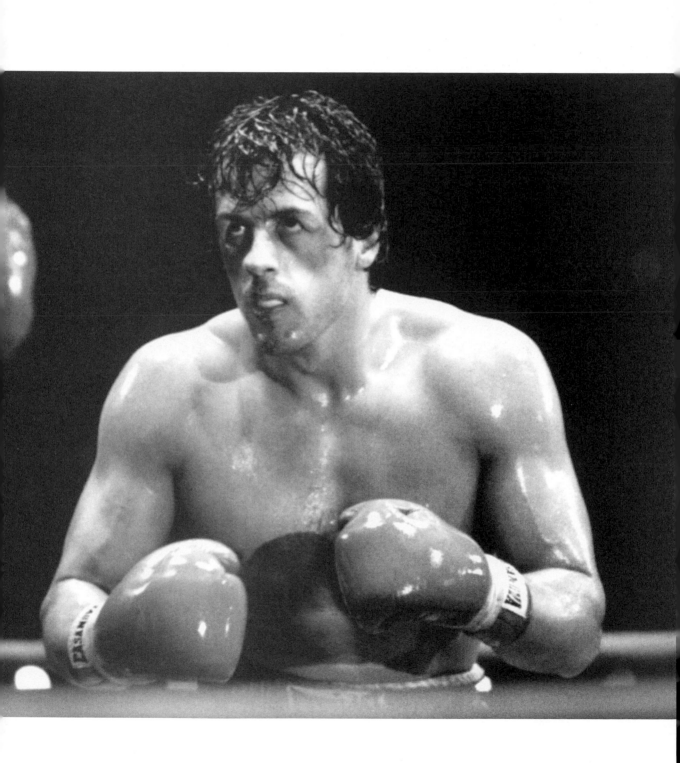

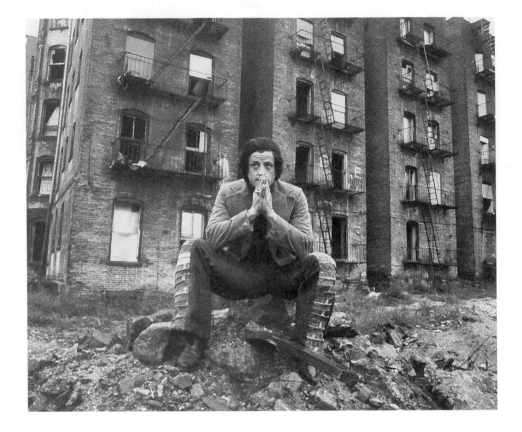

prospects in sight. My car had died, I was taking a bus to work, I even had to sell my dog, Butkus. I thought: "I may be totally wrong, but I just have to go after this. I have to believe it can happen."

It wasn't enough that the screenplay actually sold. I told the studio they could have it for free if I could play Rocky Balboa. They balked at first. The price went to nearly $360,000—which was about $359,000 more than I had ever seen. I couldn't sell. I'd been broke so long I'd gotten used to it. They finally relented and gave a total unknown a shot; for that miracle, I am forever indebted.

ABOVE: In 1976, Sly revisits the neighborhood where he was born, Hell's Kitchen in New York City. RIGHT: Sly in a recent shot.

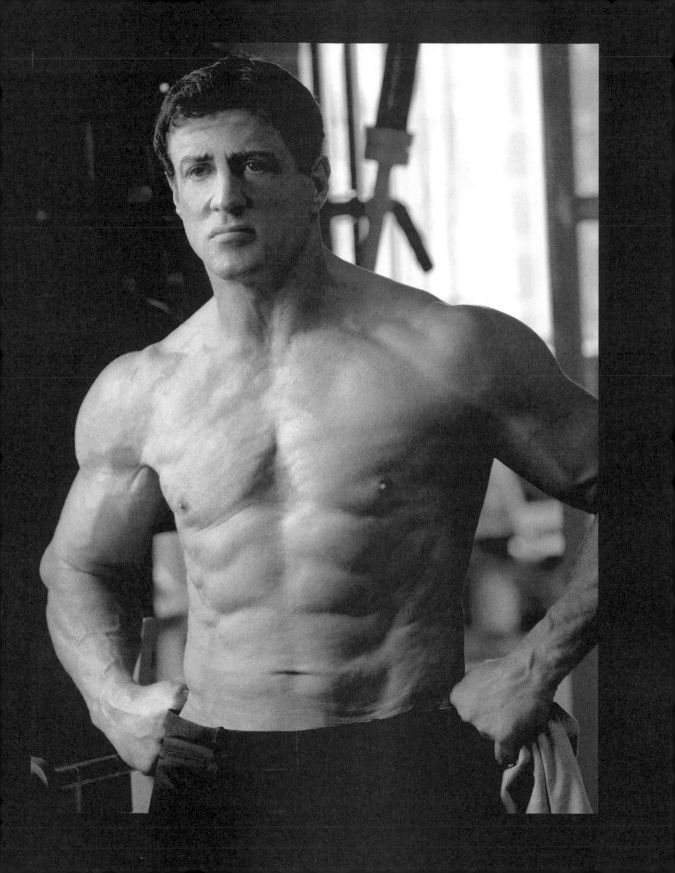

THE ONE-TWO PUNCH

Rocky was creating a buzz long before the general public ever saw it. The early private screenings around Hollywood were drawing cheers and a few standing ovations, much to my complete astonishment. Even more shocking, important people in the film industry began tracking me down instead of the other way around. I remember John Wayne introducing himself to me at one point. John Wayne! Talk about a humbling experience.

Everything felt great until a serious case of panic set in. Shortly before

QUIT SMOKING: NO IFS, ANDS, OR BUTTS

I smoked cigarettes from the time I was 13 until I was 29 and in the middle of making *Rocky*. You see me smoking in the movie, actually. Like so many millions of people, I smoked because I thought it was glamorous and a great way to look mature. Actors did it. Presidents did it. Even athletes smoked. I remember Arnold Palmer swinging a golf club with a cigarette in his hand. There used to be so much smoke at boxing matches, they'd call them "smokers." Smoking was sensual, sexy, mysterious, and—surprise, surprise—it was killing people. You certainly don't need me to tell you about the damage nicotine can do.

I'd gotten away with the habit for years, but when I really started pushing my body for *Rocky*, I knew I had to quit. When I first started training for those fight scenes with Carl Weathers, I'd start gasping after 30 seconds. It was like someone had parked a Buick on my chest. Quitting was next to impossible. I can't tell you how many times I said, "This is my last cigarette." After maybe 200 attempts, I somehow managed to go a month without one and discovered how much more I could taste and smell. In fact, that was what ultimately got me to stop. After being away from cigarettes for a while, I walked into a room where people had been smoking and I got nauseous. That sealed it.

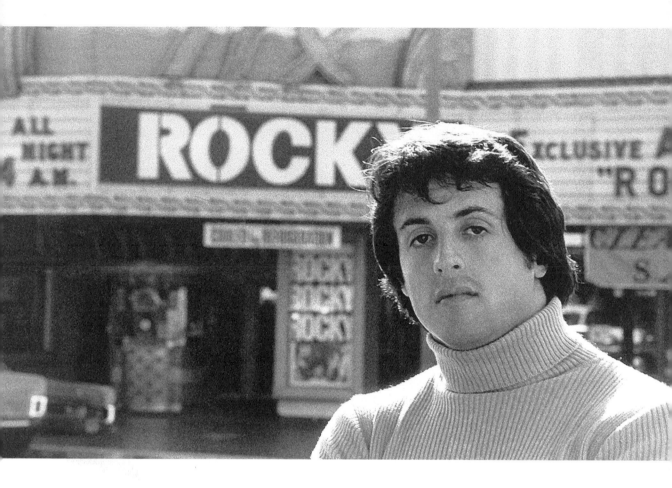

Rocky opened in a few theaters, I attended one last private screening at the Directors Guild of America. I still remember it vividly. I brought my mother and wore my new $40 suit from the May Company. Earlier screenings had been supersuccessful, but this was Hollywood. The Real Test. This audience was hard-core and sophisticated studio executives, screenwriters, and directors whose respect I so desperately wanted. But after the final credits, the theater went silent. You could hear crickets. My mother and I just sat there

ABOVE: On the cusp of fame: Rocky's first movie-house run.

until everyone left. I took a deep breath and figured the wild ride was history. But then, as we walked down the stairs to the lobby, I saw people waiting. Nearly the entire crowd, 800 strong, had gathered at the bottom of the steps to give me a tremendous ovation. I knew in that moment my whole life had changed.

The *Rocky* story is so impossible to believe, I still don't know how it happened. You go from a concept that never made any money—because nearly every boxing film had always faltered—to winning an Oscar for best picture for one of the most inexpensive studio films ever made. As the movie became a national and international hit, it felt like I was living an impossible dream.

Some of the letters I received were humbling. President Carter sent a note saying he and Rosalynn watched *Rocky* in the White House screening room and absolutely loved it. I got extraordinary letters from childhood heroes, including Kirk Douglas and William Holden. Frank Capra, the director of *It's a Wonderful Life*, said *Rocky* was a movie he wished he'd made. Even Muhammad Ali wrote me a poem:

> *You fought and you worked*
> *You're a determined guy.*
> *Rocky is great and we all love you, Sly.*
> *And if you get an Oscar, remember please do*
> *The Greatest will also get one*
> *Cause I'm prettier than you!*

Elvis asked if I'd like to come to Tennessee to screen the movie. Charlie Chaplin invited me to Switzerland. Surreal.

Once *Rocky* won Academy Awards, everyone was wondering what I would do next. I had the same question. All I knew was that I wanted to do something drastically different.

But as the 1970s drew to a close, I suddenly realized the greatest opportunity to physically alter a character was right under my nose. Why can't you follow a character as he grows? Rather than push Rocky away, I could transform him mentally and physically. For *Rocky II* not only would

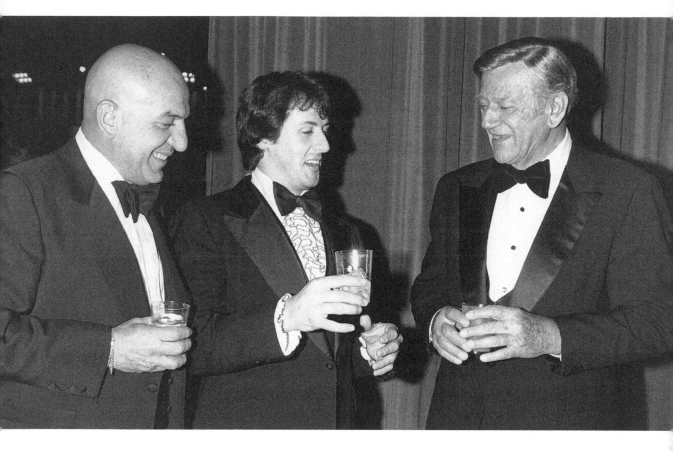

I give audiences something slightly different, I would show them that Rocky, like all of us, is a work in progress.

I'd known since I was 12 years old that the way to change your life was to change your body. I thought, why should it be any different now? Changing my body had become my secret turnaround move. For *F.I.S.T.*, the movie that followed *Rocky*, I added 35 pounds to play a union boss on the rise. For *Paradise Alley*, my next movie, it was all about "energy foods"—nuts, fruits, juices, pulverized chicken—and I got lean again.

ABOVE: Backstage with Telly Savalas and John Wayne at the Oscars in 1977.

I knew I needed guidance this time, so I summoned the body of all bodies. My hero, Steve Reeves, had retired from bodybuilding by then because of a shoulder injury, so I called on the remarkable Franco Columbu.

Franco was born on the Mediterranean island of Sardinia during World War II, and during the 1960s, he started racking up bodybuilding titles and eventually won Mr. Europe, Mr. World, Mr. Olympia, and Mr. Universe. The fitness magazines called Franco "The Sardinian Strongman."

We worked out in Franco's single-car garage in Santa Monica. It was the oddest place, mainly because he had this pet, a hostile one-winged owl. As we'd work out, the bird would glare at me, intermittently flapping that lonely wing of his, as if to say "get out." Franco was from the old school of "ground and pound" workouts. Down and dirty, nothing glamorous. But I followed his every move, 100 percent. *That included a diet of yogurt, yogurt, and, for dessert, a little more yogurt!*

The problem was, the more yogurt I ate, the slower and bulkier I got—just the opposite of my hope for a more defined character. Maybe my bones were getting stronger, but I was so bloated I felt like I'd be going the same route as the *Hindenburg*. If you'd lit a match, I would have gone up in a fireball.

Franco was definitely a tough guy. A year or so earlier, he'd shattered his leg racing with a 600-pound refrigerator full of sand on his back during the World's Strongest Man competition. Yes, it's true. Miraculously, he worked his way back and would win more bodybuilding titles. Clearly, the man knew what he was doing. But it turned out his body was just completely different than mine when it came to processing food. Yogurt slowly brought the curtain down on our working relationship.

At the end of one of our intensely competitive lifting sessions, Franco challenged me to a bench-pressing contest. Like an idiot, I accepted. Remember, this is a man who runs with a bone-crushing, 600-pound sand-filled refrigerator tied to his back for amusement.

But since we were just a month away from shooting the movie, I thought what the hell: 250, 275, 300, 315, 330 pounds. This is when your male ego should be removed from your head and left in a drawer at home. Franco Colombu to this day is considered, pound for pound, maybe the strongest bodybuilder of all time. Did I ask to be excused? Did I say I'm late for a doctor's appointment? No, I tried to beat him. So I pushed with all I had!

Bang! My pectoralis major exploded! The muscle anchored to the ribs that holds the arm in place suffered a massive tear during the lift. Tumbling off the bench, I collapsed onto my right shoulder and stared in disbelief as the ripped veins in my right arm turned my arm nearly black and doubled its size. I'm writhing on the floor, cursing my luck, trying not to black out. Maybe I was hallucinating, but I swear I could see the single-winged owl smiling and trying desperately to clap.

One hundred and sixty stitches and an attachment cable through my shoulder bone put me in dry dock for two months. That's when I was informed that a yogurt diet alone (or any other pure protein diet, for that matter) won't provide enough fiber to build muscle, especially for the kind of muscle I was using that day. It all proved to be a valuable lesson, one I can hopefully pass on to my beautiful children: *Defective owls, mega amounts of yogurt, and challenging a superhuman Sardinian is a definite formula for disaster.*

The injury actually turned out to be a very good dramatic device. The insurance company wanted to shut down production, but I convinced them it didn't matter that I couldn't use my right arm. I rewrote the end of the script so that Rocky's manager, Mickey, in a last-minute strategic move, advises Rocky to switch to southpaw (left-handed) as a way to blindside Apollo and win the fight. The plan worked. We filmed on schedule and *Rocky II* was number one in the world that year. Maybe I should've gotten badly damaged before every film. For "good luck," I mean.

THE ROAD TO RAMBO

Most actors would be pleased to be associated with one indelible character like Rocky. I've had the great fortune of being associated with two. John Rambo was an ex–Green Beret haunted by the ghosts of Vietnam, an icon of the 1980s (at least that's what *Time* magazine called him), and playing him got me in the best shape of my life.

Like Rocky, Rambo was an intensely physical role that demanded months of training each time I played him. I wanted the character's look to reflect his hard-core personality, and from the beginning that meant finding new ways to strengthen and build my body.

Fortunately, when I made *First Blood*, the first of three Rambo movies, I was already in good shape, having just completed *Rocky III*. For that film, I had really gone all out. My intention was to show how far Rocky had come since his days of struggle and strife. With success in the ring, he had practically become a one-man industry, with magazine covers and endorsement deals to prove it, and I wanted his body to reflect his superhuman status and perhaps growing egotism.

The way I trained for *Rocky III* was a bit of an overkill. I would run three miles in the morning, then go straight into 15 rounds of sparring, followed by two hours in the weight room, pushing tons of iron. Then I'd usually do 500 sit-ups before jumping rope for 10 rounds (30 minutes). I'd eat, nap, and start again. In the afternoons, I'd take another run, do some more heavy lifting, and then finish up with a long swim. It was difficult to turn off the desire to train. I'd think about it obsessively. Sometimes, I would even leave a movie or dinner party at night and drive home to work out no matter what the time—one or two in the morning, it didn't matter. This is how not to train, because when it becomes an obsession, it does much more harm than good. So I include this story only as a cautionary tale.

I was just as gung ho about my diet then, too. Most days, I'd eat little more than tuna straight out of the can for protein, a slice of burnt toast, water, and gallons of coffee. My friend John Travolta had graciously given me an espresso machine and I'd sometimes have more than 30 tiny cups of coffee a day to help speed my metabolism. It was only later that I realized I needed all that caffeine because I wasn't getting enough energy from food.

All that effort certainly appeared to be working. I went from having 14 percent body fat to around 2.8 percent. (In those days, Mr. Olympia would have measured in around 4 percent; the average guy around 18–20 percent.) And at a gaunt 161 pounds, I was leaner than ever but certainly not healthier. The International Federation of Bodybuilders named me the "Body of the

RIGHT: While training for Rocky III, *Sly reduced his body fat to 2.8 percent.*

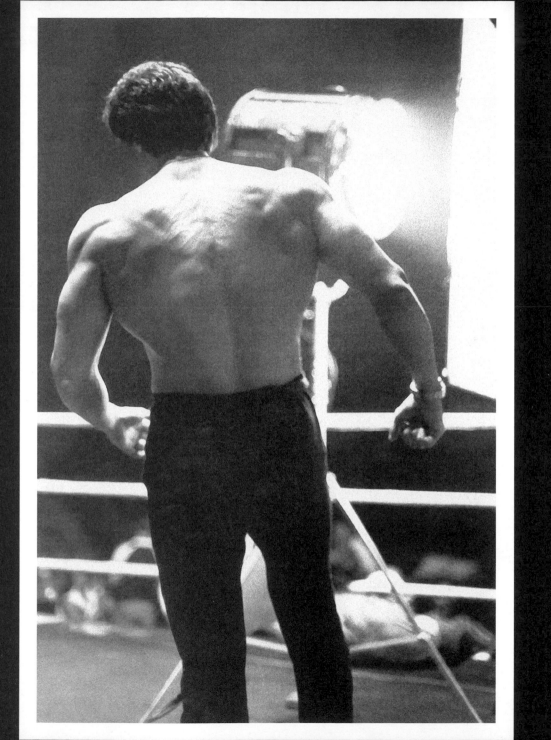

80s," an amazing honor for a nonprofessional. One newspaper described my body as "surrealistically fit." No doubt about it, I almost had veins in my hair.

I was under a fair amount of stress during that time because I was also directing *Rocky III*, and I looked forward to letting up a bit after the movie wrapped. Since I was merely going to cowrite and star in *First Blood*, I thought, hey, this should feel like a vacation.

The script for *First Blood* had been floating around Hollywood for a long time, and many prominent actors and directors, including Clint Eastwood, Steve McQueen, Nick Nolte, Michael Douglas, Al Pacino, and Robert De Niro, had passed on it for one reason or another. But I connected to the Rambo story. Plus, they most likely ran out of actors, so their misfortune was my good luck. I got to play a character that touched a chord with audiences around the world and crossed cultural lines.

I believe what really made Rambo a success, though, was that the character spoke with his body. The original cut of *First Blood* ran almost three hours and was full of orations about the plight of America's neglected soldiers. It was a completely different film. Rambo even dies in the original version. But by editing the movie down to 97 minutes, and losing almost all the dialogue, we created a man who was completely emotional and physical. It turned out that words were pointless with Rambo. He expressed himself clearly with sinewy catlike moves and haunted eyes that said everything about the estrangement and abandonment he felt.

Making Rambo a purely physical creature had major implications for me, especially once the studio started pushing for a sequel. In the first movie, John Rambo looked fit but he certainly wasn't a bodybuilder type. There was none of that narcissism. He was a regular athletic guy whose power was very much under control, even subdued. He was practically Zen. Some people talk about the violence in the movie, but Rambo here isn't so much a killing machine as someone who fought back only in self-defense. The only regret about playing Rambo was my borderline insane choice to play the character in a damp, moth-eaten tank top during the coldest Canadian winter in a hundred years.

As you might have guessed, making *First Blood* wasn't a vacation at all. My workouts were less intense than on *Rocky III*, but the actual film-ing was tougher. I opted to do many of my own stunts, so I was constantly leaping from ledges and scuttling over roots and rocks. Shooting the scene in which Rambo jumps from a cliff and falls through trees, I landed the wrong way and cracked two ribs, leaving me in the kind of agony I hadn't experienced since I was forced to eat raw oysters as a six-year-old.

As with *Rocky*, I saw each Rambo sequel as an opportunity to change physically. I couldn't just come back every time looking like the same guy. I wanted the challenge, because a real challenge that intimidates you is the only thing that will bring out your best.

Getting into shape for *Rambo: First Blood II* meant pushing to new limits. We needed a ferocious look to match a plot that was equally pumped up.

In the story, Rambo had been in a military prison and breaking rocks, so his arms had to be powerful and hard. Months before production began, I got into an extremely intense training regimen, and as the shoot got closer, I put myself on a repetitive high-protein diet that consisted mainly of chicken, greens, and occasionally beets. On weekends I'd lighten up a bit, and maybe even have some ice cream, but come Monday, it was back to the bare minimum.

Exercise was a far too intensive six-day-a-week deal, sometimes two times a day. But thankfully we've learned with workout programs that *more* is *not* necessarily *better*, and in many cases, too much pumping and grunting can destroy positive results by leaving your body in a constant state of exhaustion. Perhaps it was overly ambitious, but I wanted to take John Rambo, a character that in the original movie had been in good shape, and turn him into a physical specimen even bodybuilders would appreciate. For me, it wasn't just about preparing for a role, this had become a personal contest of the highest order. How far could I push myself? I wondered.

The workout routines were usually what we call supersets and split sets, with 15 to 20 sets of exercises targeting every part of the body. If you're not into weight training, this was hard-core. I literally lived in the gym. Then I would come home at night and before bed I'd do 200 sit-ups,

250 push-ups, 100 chin-ups. *Again, this was far more work than necessary to have gotten the desired results* (more later on a scientific approach that will produce dramatic results without demanding so much of your free time).

Those big *Rambo II* brushstrokes signaled the beginning of a new kind of über–action hero. Yes, we'd had physically strong movie heroes before—John Wayne, Steve McQueen, Kirk Douglas—but now people were viewing Rambo, with his bandana, gun, and bandoleer, as a kind of personification of an American war machine. I wasn't sure how I felt about it, but that didn't matter. The character was taking on a life of its own.

It was an interesting time for me personally, especially once Ronald Reagan announced he was a Rambo fan. President Reagan had a habit of telling jokes to technicians over his open microphone as he prepared to address the nation. In June 1985, before a live speech from the Oval Office following the release of 39 American hostages in Lebanon, he said, "After seeing *Rambo* last night, I know what to do the next time this happens." The comment leaked out and by summer's end, after the president referenced the movie again, Rambo was suddenly a school of thought. He'd become an "ism."

In a way, it was flattering that people in such lofty positions were paying so much attention, even if that attention wasn't always positive. But the funny thing is, I never saw Rambo as a political figure! The character was completely neutral, completely apathetic to policies. To me, he was like an American tragedy. He was a fallen hero and underdog whose only dream was to be loved and appreciated by his country. We built him, trained him, then discarded him, leaving him unwanted and homeless. I had a lot of time to contemplate Rambo's impact on society, which came as a total surprise, because Rambo was being touted as a failure in the making. But I have to hand it to the producers, because they took a gigantic chance on a "jinxed" and controversial project. It had been passed around Hollywood for years, simply because no one could figure out how to crack the "bleakness" and depressing ending of the story, where Rambo must die.

But I didn't think it was such a difficult problem because the story embodied almost the same

RIGHT: With Ronald Reagan at the White House.

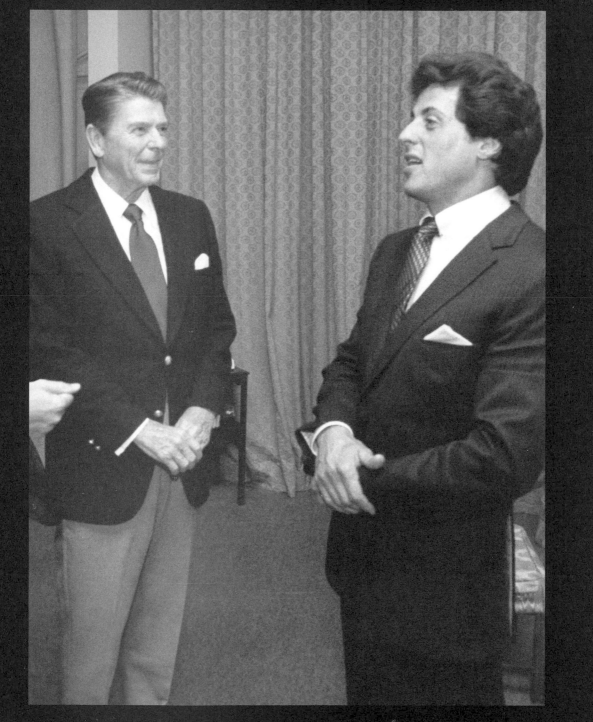

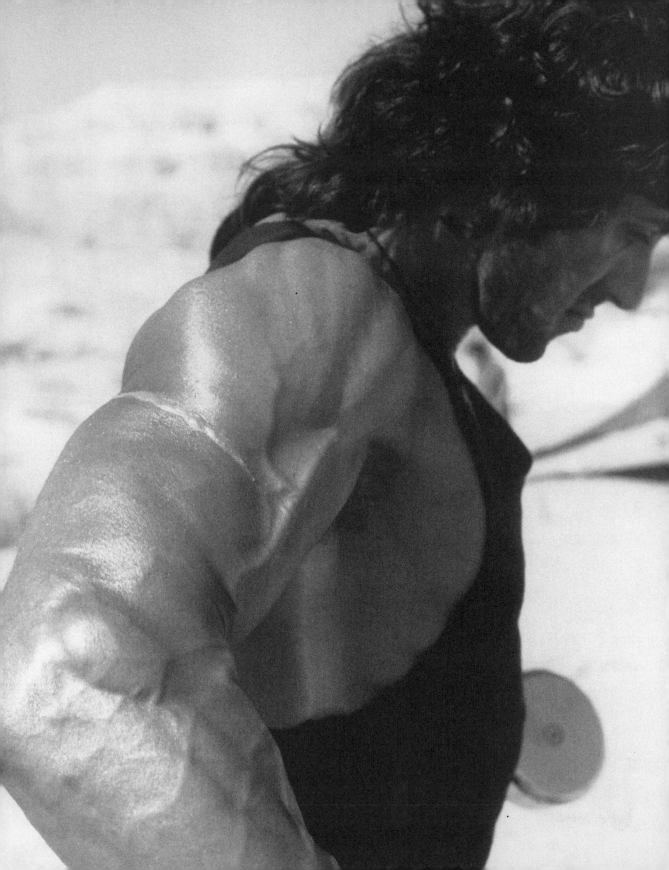

philosophy as this book: People want to live up to their ideals. People need to believe *tomorrow can be better than yesterday and today.*

SAND AND SWEAT

At 1,320 feet below sea level, the Dead Sea on the border between Israel and Jordan is the lowest point on earth. The sun scorches the surrounding desert landscape without a hint of rain for more than 330 days a year, and midday temperatures can soar to 130 degrees. This extreme environment proved to be a fitting backdrop for *Rambo III*, the most intense moviemaking experience of my life.

Rambo had become such a phenomenon by 1988 that I had to work hard to keep up with him. The movie itself was the most ambitious Rambo of them all—now our hero was going into Afghanistan to confront the menacing Russians—and I felt I needed a physique that matched that gargantuan scale. We hadn't seen the wandering warrior in four years, so when he is revealed for the first time, he appears to have grown in strength, which was not so much an opportunity to show off but, rather, a not-so-subtle message that you're never too old to keep improving.

Rambo III conveniently coincided with the end of *Rocky IV*, in which I'd pumped myself up to box with Dolph Lundgren, who played Rocky's superhuman Russian opponent. But I knew I'd have to be in better shape for this one.

The challenge wasn't just about getting into great shape. By that point, I knew how to do that. The trick was *maintaining* the look. In most movies, you have to remain at the character's exact weight and appearance for months at a time. I decided to add 15 pounds of muscle from where I'd been in *Rambo II* and went from 163 pounds to around 178, 180. Now I needed to stay that way. Those desert conditions certainly didn't make it easy. Memos were posted around the set reminding everyone to drink 20 to 30 cups of water a day and to stay out of the midday sun. To beat the heat, I'd wake up at five-thirty in the morning, and sometimes it

LEFT: Training in the desert for Rambo III, *where temperatures averaged 118 degrees.*

would already be 95 degrees. Soon enough, a camel with a large family of flies perched on its lower lip would pick me up to take me to my "gym," which was just a few dumbbells in the sand.

Thinking back on it, I was slightly insane for what I put myself through. Most mornings, I'd do 40 sets of exercises and 10 to 15 repetitions of each. Everyone has a body part that is on average stronger than the rest; mine is my back. I would do pull-downs with 275 pounds of weight at a time when I only weighed 180. They literally had to strap me to the bench so I wouldn't snap in two!

But I saved the real work for the abdominals. I convinced myself that it's one thing to get big arms or a big chest, but the midsection tells the real story. At the time, I believed it, but I've come to learn you can be in fantastic health and be incredibly fit and not have anything close to a six-pack, not even a one-pack. *So don't worry about it*. Not that you could have convinced me back then. Still lost in the bodybuilding dark ages, I turned to archaic training methods like hanging from an old-fashioned wall rack while kicking my legs above my head. Or I'd suspend myself upside down with weights in my hands and jackknife my body straight back up. Again, this is far too extreme, and at the time I didn't know any better. After thousands of years of man doing a carnivalesque array of exercises, some even life-threatening, modern fitness experts have finally figured it out, measuring how to get the most by doing the least. *Overtraining wasted thousands of hours of my life.*

From a production standpoint, *Rambo III* was a massive undertaking, and to keep my focus, I made sure I had all the right tools at the ready. I had an 18-piece gym set up at our Dead Sea accommodations. And to keep my diet consistent, I ate chicken and a green vegetable seven days a week, twice a day. I'm proud to say that by the end of the shoot, I nearly had grown an attractive layer of feathers.

I also traveled around in an armored Jeep, but that wasn't a luxury at all. We got a ton of death threats during the three months we spent in Israel, but I didn't think for a moment it was political. I thought for sure it was most likely a critic who'd seen my last several films. We

RIGHT: Training for Rambo III.

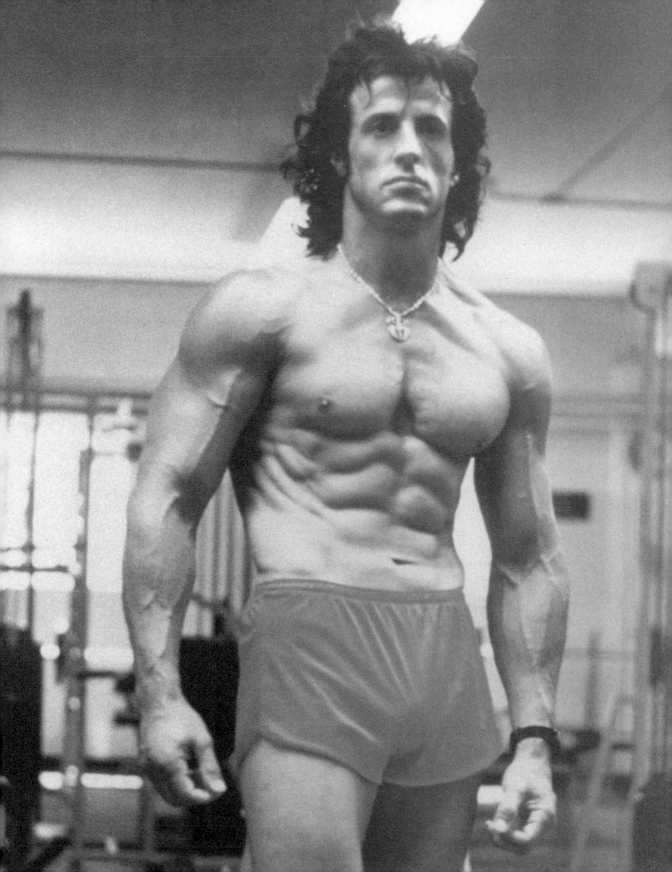

even got word from the CIA about an Iranian plot to kidnap me, and we wound up bringing in Ariel Sharon, the former Israeli defense minister and future prime minister, to advise us. One afternoon when shots rang out near the hotel, security whisked me into a safe room in the hotel basement. I remained there for over an hour. It was hot, dark, and depressing, as only hotel basements can be. So to make it more comfortable, they sent out for food, and what did they bring back? You guessed it: a desert chicken sandwich served on bread that doubled for wall board. Truthfully, at this point in my diet, a sniper's bullet would have been easier to swallow.

Rambo III was made before the days of computer-generated effects, so we had to do everything for real—rappelling out of helicopters, lying under a moving tank, running through explosions. The closest call came when a French Puma helicopter banked the wrong way during the shooting of a fight and nearly decapitated me and one of the stuntmen. I have such admiration for the men and women who do this type of stunt work for a living, and I owe them a great deal. But I owe a horse my life. Pound for pound the most dangerous stunt I've ever been involved with was in *Rambo III*, where Rambo is invited to play buzkashi, which is the most dangerous game in the world; the idea is to grab the body of a 75-pound sheep and gallop several hundred yards and drop it in the "circle of triumph." Sounds easy enough, except for the 20 other horsemen doing their very best to smash you into the earth. Even the competing horses revel in the prospect of tumbling someone to the dust and delivering a well-placed kick. The danger of playing on sandy soil with its many hidden sharp-edged rocks was a formula for a deadly accident. Several horsemen went down rupturing spleens, another shattered both hips, and a third rider landed so hard that he went temporarily blind for several hours. My horse, a magnificent and fearless Andalusian stallion, carried me through hours of this insane stunt.

Interestingly enough, after all that sweat, punishment, and chicken, after the near-death experiences and those close-call explosions, Rambo was nearly undone by a petite woman in a Chanel suit. In *Rambo III*, the Russians are depicted as America's worst nightmare, the red menace of the Evil Empire. Their involvement in Afghanistan was portrayed as Russia's

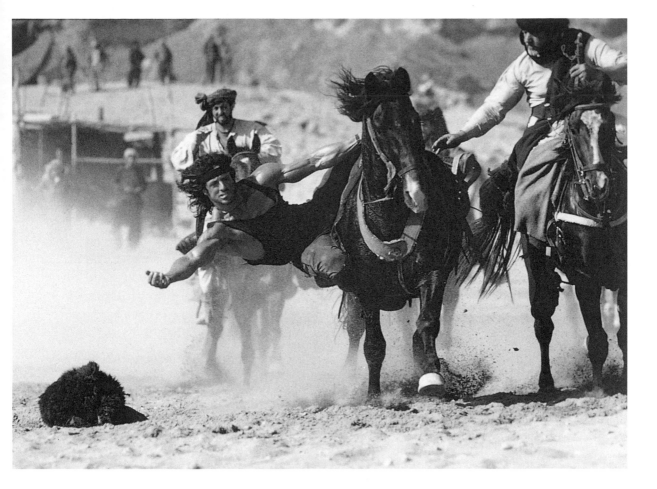

Vietnam. But by the time the film premiered, the Soviet army announced the withdrawal of its troops from Afghanistan. And to make matters worse, there on every station in the world was Mikhail Gorbachev kissing Nancy Reagan on the cheek, so by the time the big Russian had unpuckered, the Soviets were now our new best friends and Rambo was decreed to be a red-baiting, right-wing killing machine designed to

ABOVE: Playing what is considered the most dangerous game in the world, buzkashi.

show our new loving buddies from the east in a bad light. So much for mixing drama and politics. Truthfully, if Gorby could have postponed that kiss for another two weeks, we would have been home free. Maybe it was payback for besting the Russian Beast, Ivan Drago, in *Rocky IV*. Yes, that must've been it.

THE ROLE OF A LIFETIME

Imagine this scenario if you can. You are flying in an airplane over the United States of America and as the flight attendant refills your water glass, you casually glance out the window to some distant city lights below. High wispy clouds are whipping by at 500 miles an hour, and as they break apart, the insanity of your life suddenly comes into sharp focus. You could be over Cleveland or Tucson or Slippery Rock, Pennsylvania. In fact, you could be 35,000 feet above Hong Kong or Athens or Lima, Peru, and the situation would still be the same: almost everyone down there knows who you are.

You might think I'd be jaded by now. But, the older I get, the more I realize what a miracle this life is.

It would be very easy to lose perspective, but I'm blessed to have a family that keeps me focused on the things that really matter. My wife, Jennifer, and my children are continued sources of pride, and our home is a grounding force for me.

The other thing that's kept me sane through the years is the gym. It's been my refuge as long as I can remember. For instance, when I lived in Miami in the early 1990s, I had a gym in the house and it was an excellent place to relieve stress and clarify my thoughts. I was on the verge of turning 50, an age when many people start to slow down. I certainly wasn't ready for that and exercise was my way of gathering momentum rather than losing it. This wasn't the same punishing regimen I'd followed before. I started practicing yoga and tai chi and focused more on smoothing out than on bulking up. My workouts went from 25 hours a week to three or four, which gave me time to pursue other interests.

I don't think it's a coincidence

RIGHT: Directing traffic in Cop Land *after a gain of 40 pounds.*

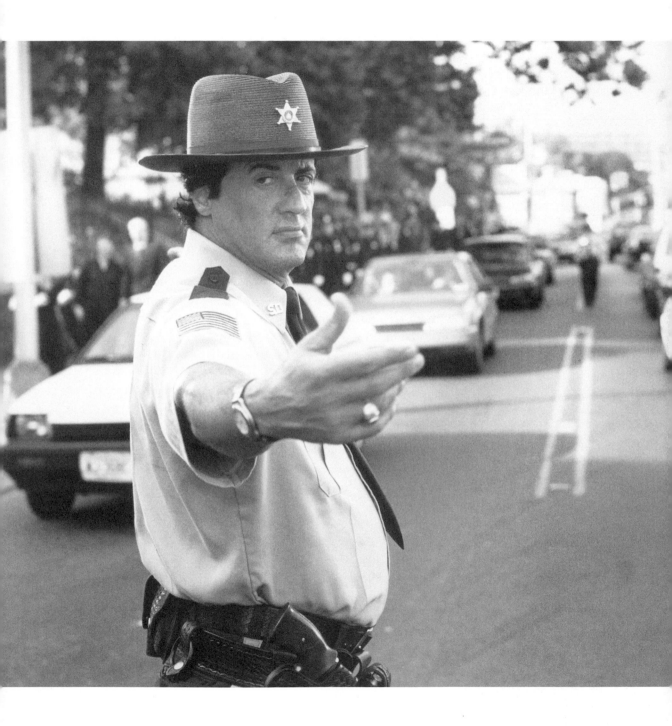

that simplifying my workout coincided with a whole new outlook. For many years, I was incredibly competitive with myself. Each new project, every new film had to be another test in some way. As good as things were, they would always be better next time. I know I'm not alone in falling into that trap. So many people think happiness is always just on the horizon. The next job, the next raise, the next car . . . *that's* the one that's going to make the difference. That next vacation's going to do it or else that next gadget or house or kid. Unfortunately, life does not work that way. You can get all those things, multiply them by a hundred thousand, and still feel unfulfilled.

Part of the turnaround that has put me in good stead these last 10 years was my role in a 1996 movie called *Cop Land*. Gaining 40 pounds to play a small-town New Jersey sheriff, I was able to let go of some very old thoughts about body image. I actually had fun packing on the pounds and was amazed how the extra weight changed people's reactions to me. People approached me without trepidation and I lost the edge of aggressiveness that sometimes accompanied my intense movie workouts. I'd gotten in touch with something very special that was close to my heart, acid reflux. Just kidding. Actually, I'm not: it was one of the many problems I acquired when I gained weight. Some of the other *acquaintances* I made were heart palpitations, elevated blood pressure, back problems, even flatter feet.

Since *Cop Land*, my professional work has taken a backseat to greater pleasures in my life. This may sound odd, but I've learned to enjoy the art of leisure time without feeling guilty. I've found incredible happiness in my marriage. And I can't begin to describe the joy of waking up every morning to my little ones, Sophia, Sistine, and Scarlett.

I've also developed a healthy lifestyle that keeps me feeling better than ever with less effort than you can imagine. I rarely spend more than three and a half hours a week in the gym, and I actually enjoy food instead of obsessing over it. I weigh almost 20 pounds more than when I did *Rocky*, but I've never felt physically stronger.

Life is like juggling in the dark. It's impossible not to make mistakes. You're going to drop the ball sometimes. It's the only way you learn. No one beats life. Everybody battles fears, temptations, and personal shortcomings every single day.

How you treat your body is a central determining force in how this one precious life of yours will turn out. As I see it, when it comes to health and fitness, you can go in three directions: up, down, or sideways. You can define yourself by the devils inside your head and by a body you've never really loved, or you can travel a new path, be satisfied with your present life, and make peace with the past.

BIG LIKE ME: THE GAINS AND PAINS OF COP LAND

In 1997, I starred with Robert De Niro, Harvey Keitel, and Ray Liotta in a film about a downtrodden small-town New Jersey cop who uncovers corruption in the NYPD. *Cop Land* got good reviews, but most people remember it for how overweight I was in it. The director insisted that my character, Sheriff Freddy Heflin, be as soft-bellied as he was sad. I decided to play him like a human turtle—slow, unsteady, terrified of the world. As soon as I read the script, I knew I'd have to gain weight. Lots of weight.

Over the course of three months, I packed on 40 pounds and went from a 31-inch waist to a $39^1/_2$-inch waist. In the process, I learned a tremendous amount about the physiology and psychology of being overweight.

First, I saw how easy it is to put on pounds. I'd wake up in the morning and do nothing. No exercise, no stretching, no problem. I'd head over to a place called the Royal Canadian Pancake House—after a while, I started calling it "the trough"—and eat whatever I wanted. Some days it would be five pancakes, some days 10, whatever I could handle, and I always topped it with mountains of whipped cream and washed it down with chocolate milk.

These pancakes were so big, you could put an axle in them and drive home. God, I miss those days. Then again, I don't.

For a while, I loved bulking up. I actually had fun. After decades of being conscientious about my weight, it was a fantastic relief to let go.

But then the check came.

I developed sciatica, heart palpitations, debilitating acid reflux, digestion problems, and headaches. My cholesterol and blood pressure levels were astronomically high. Those afternoon energy lapses soon turned into full-fledged exhaustion; as a special added bonus, I got a full-blown case of sleep apnea. In one year I'd gone from best abs to the worst adenoids.

As soon as production wrapped, I went on my version of the Atkins diet, which was about 80 percent protein and the rest just good fats: Nuts, avocado, olive oil, things like that. I got back into a regular cardio routine and started weight training again. I lost 40 pounds in 60 days without killing myself. Muscle memory is an amazing thing.

I finally understood the uncomfortable situations being physically overweight puts people into, which is the reason I wanted to do this book.

THE SLY MOVES CHALLENGE

If this were a movie, we would cue the theme song right about now. You're about to regain control of your life by taking charge of the things that matter most—the way you eat, the way you treat your body, the way you go after your dreams.

It really doesn't matter where you are or what shape you're in or even how long you've let things slide. Take this as an opportunity to fly higher than you ever have before and know that your life can start improving the moment you turn the page.

My guess is you wouldn't be reading this book unless you were ready to make some profound changes. That's truly exciting, and I want you to know I support you all the way. Having heard my story, you know I've had my ups and downs. But you've also seen how the fire inside prevails even in the face of seemingly impossible odds.

Now it's time to decide how far you want to go. I'm about to share a lifetime of lessons about living better. It all begins with the mind, then the body, and from there, the sky's the limit. Just make me one promise: Never *ever* let anybody tell you you're too weak, too heavy, too small, too old, too *anything*. Wake up the sleeping giant and show the world what you're really capable of achieving.

The bell just rang. It's time to take your best shot!

★

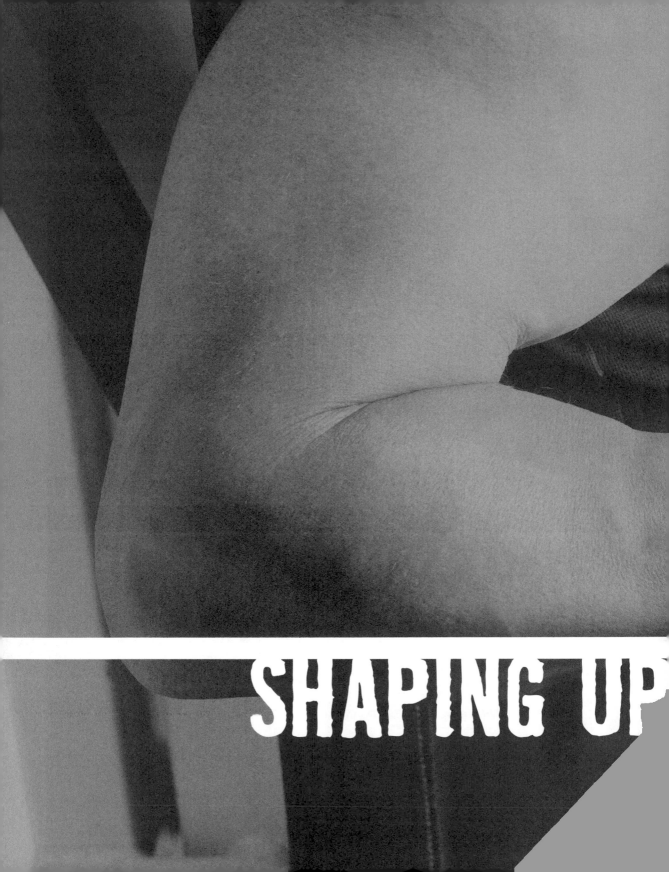

SHAPING UP

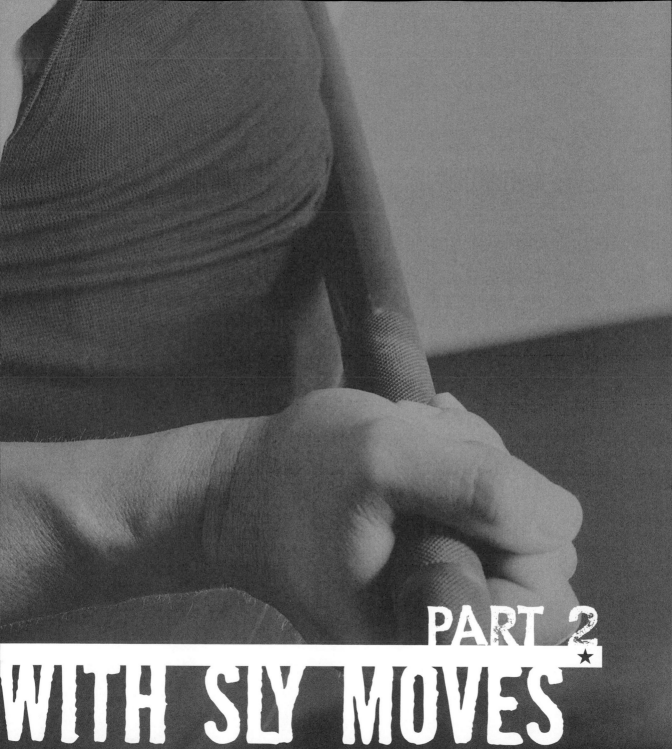

PART 2
★

WITH SLY MOVES

Wherever I go, I meet people who want to know how to manage their weight, boost their energy levels, and generally get the fires going again in life. It doesn't matter how intelligent or wealthy or famous they are, the question is always the same: "How can *I* get in good shape?!"

I feel better and stronger now than ever, so why can't you? The program that follows is the most practical way I know to respond to all those who've asked me about health and fitness over the years. The exercise routines I'm about to describe all really work—whether you're a scrawny 13-year-old kid like I was or a 75-year-old who wants to give life one more swift kick in the ass. That said, I've also included a separate set of workouts specifically tailored for women.

Later in this section, I'll show you exactly how to structure your workouts, day by day, week by week, for years to come, whether you're a beginner, a weekend athlete, or a serious gym fanatic. And as you'll discover in the next section, diet is every bit as significant as breathing when it comes to staying strong and living long.

I realize that for some of you, beginning this program—or even just stepping foot inside a gym—will be a major stretch. You're in good company. Many people out there view dumbbells and treadmills the way early man viewed solar eclipses: as something otherworldly, and frightening.

The truth is, most gyms aren't full of bodybuilders anymore. You have soccer moms and Nascar dads and Nintendo boys and girls. There are teachers and accountants and delivery-room nurses. Everybody in the gym has a different story and yet they all have the same goal: to become better than they were before.

After lifting for more than four decades, I can honestly say that if you have a plan (which I'm about to give you), set reachable goals (I'll help you there, too), and progress slowly (that's the easy part), working with weights can *and will* become one of the great pleasures of your life. Best of all, the workouts won't even take much time. One hour three times a week is all that's required to get into the best shape of your life. That's it! That's all it takes to radically improve your physique.

Still not convinced? Maybe these sobering facts will help. Did you know that as early as our late twenties, muscle tissue gradually begins to disappear as a natural part of the aging process? Think about that. By the time you hit 30, *you're slowly starting to fade out*. When you lose muscle, the number of calories you require on a daily basis decreases and it becomes much easier to gain weight. That explains the paunch of middle age.

Let me tell you a few things that exercising can do, then tell me this isn't worth it: Exercise builds new muscle, strengthens bones, ligaments, and tendons. It increases coordination, agility, and does wonders for confidence and energy levels. Exercise can improve your mood, increase your stamina, calm your nerves, and give a turbo boost to your love life, career, and future goals.

I could go on and on but suffice it to say that you can't live a completely fulfilled life without some form of regular exercise. I honestly believe that. For one thing, *nobody* ever lost weight and kept it off without engaging in at least a little physical activity. And while walking and cycling and jogging are noble pursuits, that sort of aerobic conditioning doesn't preserve your muscles. If it did, long-distance runners would be the strongest people on earth. Let me say it again: there's absolutely no substitute for weight resistance training. *None. Not if you want to feel and look better than you have in years.*

Even if you're starting from scratch, even if you don't know your latissimus dorsi muscle from a doughnut, you're not as far from feeling good and getting major results as you might think. As soon as you lift your first weight, you're improving your chances of living a longer life, and feeling better than you did two minutes before you opened this book.

THE MOVES

Here are the tried-and-true gym exercises that have kept me going and growing as long as I can remember. I promise you'll see results after a few short weeks. These step-by-step instructions will guide you through the moves and help you avoid certain classic mistakes. I've also included some thoughts on each one. Following the descriptions, you'll find my suggested drills for working out. Once you pick the plan that's right for you, you'll know exactly what to do every time you're at the gym.

Again, I realize this might be a little intimidating to you if you're new to weight training. I completely understand. My advice for beginners is to run through these moves for the first time with a fitness trainer or an experienced friend. And use weights that you are comfortable with, and that are right for your fitness level. It's certainly not essential but it's a great way to feel at ease on some of these odd-looking machines. Remember, I want you to enjoy everything you do in the gym. *Have fun with it, expect to make some mistakes, and, above all, prepare to become that person you always wanted to be.*

★ CARDIO WARM-UP ★

The Move: Using the cardio machine of your choice, get your heart rate up to between 120 and 140 beats per minute. Work up to an intensity level of 8 out of 10. One of the best is the rowing machine. Super for the buttocks.

Time: 5 minutes.

The Sly Report: Cardio work is very personal and, personally, I hate doing it. That's the truth. So I tend to use elliptical machines, which lessen the impact on my knees and hips and are more fun to use. If you walk on a treadmill, set it at a steep incline. Like the rowing machine, the other ultimate cardio workout is the VersaClimber. Five minutes on that metallic monster will curl your eyelashes.

TIP
Change machines often if it feels like it's getting monotonous.

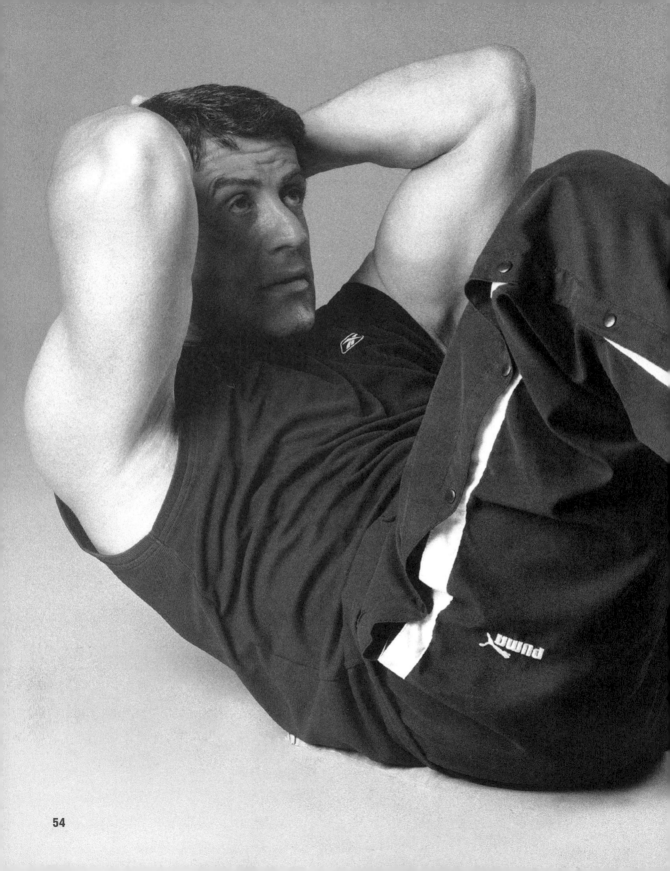

54

★ FLOOR CRUNCHES ★
(abdominals)

The Move: Lie flat on your back with your knees bent and feet on the floor. Hold your hands behind your head and roll your upper torso forward as your knees come up toward your elbows. At the top of the crunch, consciously squeeze the abdominal muscles before slowly lowering back for the next crunch. Exhale as you come up, inhale on the way back down.

Sets: 2 sets of 5, 10, or 15; work your way up to 30.

The Sly Report: Crunches are much more effective than regular sit-ups because they specifically target your upper abdominal muscles rather than your hip muscles. If you're not used to them, they can cause soreness a day or two later, but it's a "cool" soreness. A badge of honor.

TIP
If floor crunches are too tough in the beginning, start on the gym's crunch machine.

TIP
Resist the temptation to pull on your neck when you're doing crunches.

★ TWISTING CRUNCHES ★
(abdominals)

The Move: Lie on the floor with your hands behind your head, your knees bent, and feet comfortably off the ground. Exhale and curl your upper body forward, rotating your elbow towards the opposite knee.

Sets: 2 sets of 5, 10, or 15; work your way up to 30.

The Sly Report: Fortunately for you, I'm not recommending you get a kid to pound on your stomach while you're doing them, like I did in those scenes from *Rocky II*. Twisting crunches target the obliques and upper abdominals, with some secondary benefits for the lower abs. People don't realize when they "throw out" their back, it's often because of weak abs. These muscles are essential for lower back strength and good posture.

★ HANGING RAISES ★
(abdominals)

The Move: Rest your elbows in the elbow slings or on the support pads (if you're using the gym's dip station or hanging chair). Lean back slightly and slowly draw your knees toward your chest as far as possible. Return to the starting position and repeat.

Sets: 2 sets of 10.

The Sly Report: Incredible exercise for your midsection. Doing it early in your routine gets the exercise juices going and charges you up for the tougher work to come.

TIP

I try to lock the knees and roll my stomach up. If you pull in and roll back instead of lifting the legs straight, you will get a lot more out of this exercise.

★ BROOMSTICK TWISTS ★
(abdominals)

The Move: Set an incline bench with ankle supports at a 45-degree angle. Sit upright on the bench and secure your feet under the supports. Hold a broomstick behind your head and across your shoulders, supported by your outstretched arms. Twist left and right on the axis of the stick, feeling the burn at your core.

Sets: 3 sets of 10.

The Sly Report: This one gave me the best abs of my life. Later, it really helped get me chiseled for *Rambo II* and *Rambo III*. I've been using this beauty for years. The secret is the combination of incline and twist, which creates unrelenting contractions that shape what trainers now like to call the "core," a set of muscles that includes the lower back, the glutes, the hip flexors, and the mini–mountain range that runs from the abs to the obliques. A powerful core is a kind of anchor that lets you throw farther, swing harder, reach higher, and perform better, especially as you get older. So go ahead: stick it!

TIP
It's not a sit-up, so don't bend forward. This is all about the twist.

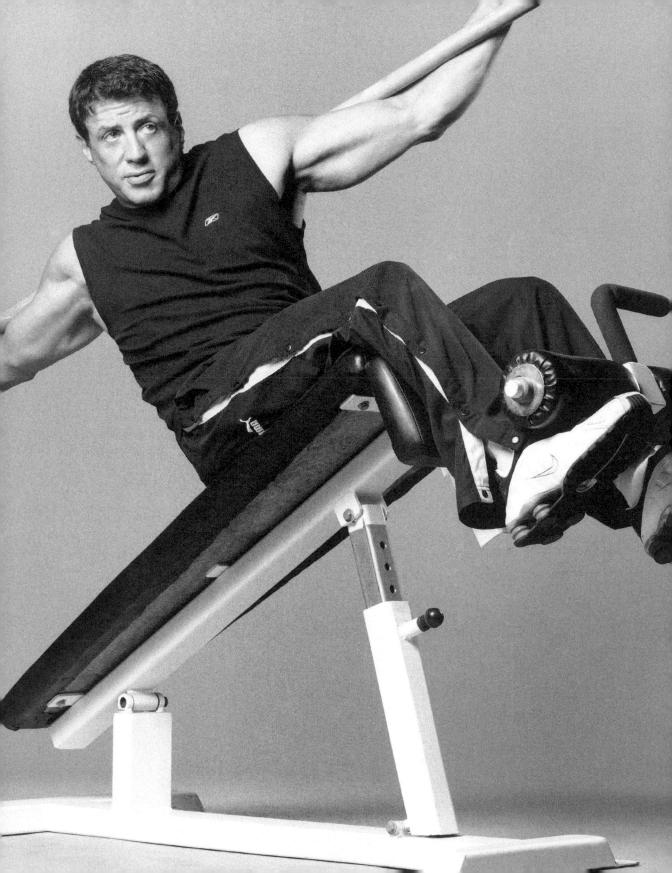

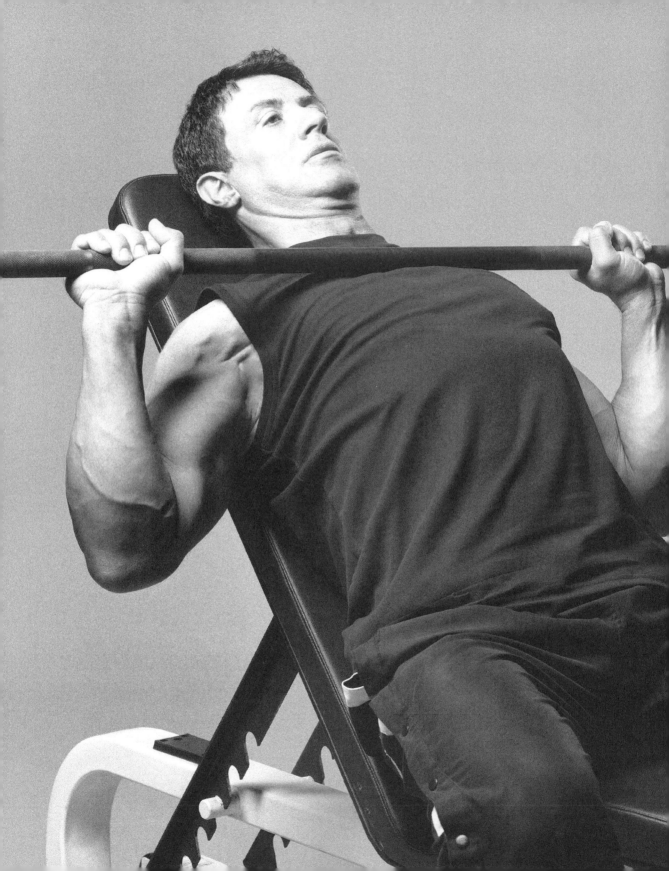

★ INCLINE BENCH PRESS ★
(chest)

The Move: Set an incline bench at an angle between 45 and 60 degrees. Lie back and take an overhand grip on a barbell with your hands more than shoulder-width apart. Inhale as you bring the bar down across the top of your chest. Exhale as you press up, fully extending your arms.

Sets: 1 light warm-up, then 3 sets of 10.

The Sly Report: A classic pectoral workout, it's great for overall symmetry. Lifting on the incline builds a flatter, almost plate-like chest, like a gymnast's, rather than that bulky bodybuilder's chest, which will cause you to be mistaken for an escaped silverback gorilla. The flatter look is more elegant and athletic, and as you age, it holds up better. For proof, look at some of our most famous aging bodybuilders. That pumped-up chest of youth now resembles collapsed feed bags.

TIP

It's essential to hear your breath as you're pressing up. Don't be modest. Breathe loud and breathe proud! It lets people around you know you're alive.

★ INCLINE BENCH ★ DUMBBELL FLYS
(chest)

The Move: Lying back on an incline bench with dumbbells in each hand, bring the weights directly overhead, arms fully extended, palms facing each other. From this starting position, lower the dumbbells out to your sides, your arms stretching wide. You'll feel the stretch across your rib cage into your arms. As you bring the weights back up, follow the natural arc back to the top, finishing overhead with the dumbbells touching.

Sets: 2 sets of 8, maximum.

The Sly Report: This is a phenomenal pectoral workout. Take your time and control your speed. I like to set the bench at a 45-degree angle, but you can go lower than that if it's more comfortable.

TIP

Don't extend too far past the shoulder joint at the bottom of the exercise. Always keep the tension on.

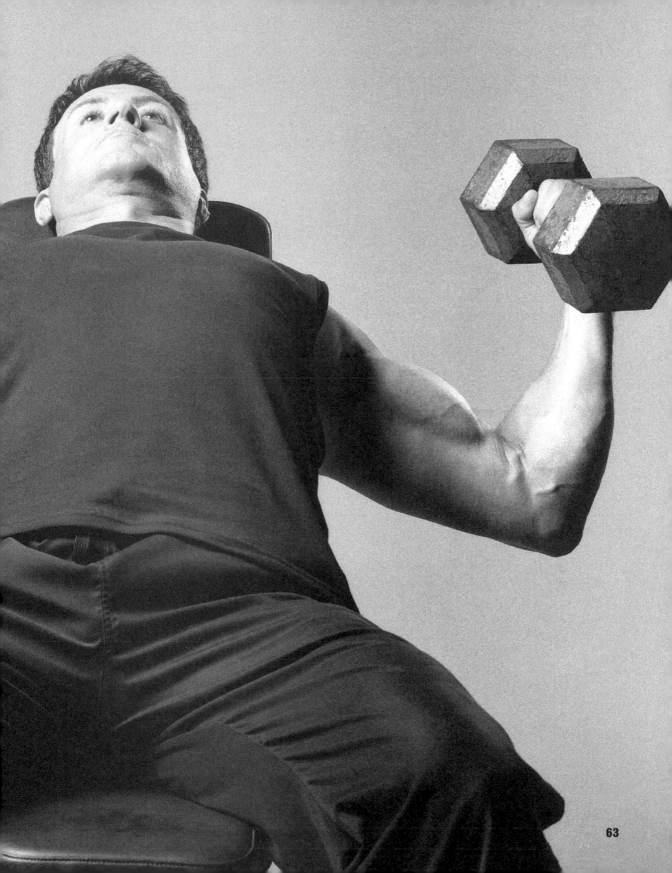

★ WIDE-ARM PUSH-UPS ★
(chest)

The Move: Assume the classic push-up position but extend your hands out about 10 inches from your shoulders. Keeping your body in a straight line and your eyes forward, push up until your arms are fully extended. Slowly lower yourself until your torso almost touches the floor and then push up again. Exhale as you press up, inhale on the way down.

Sets: 2 sets of 10; work your way up to 25.

The Sly Report: Don't worry. You won't see one-armed push-ups on this list. Wide-arm push-ups are all you need. They work the triceps and address the upper and outer portion of the chest, which get very little workout in everyday life. It's a very good move for building strength *and* fantastic triceps.

TIP
The first few times, you may only be able to manage two or three of these. But stick with it. As you build your strength with other exercises, these get easier. When you're just starting out, it helps to lift your rear end as you push up. Do that until you can maintain a straighter line.

★ BENT-OVER ★ RUNNERS
(shoulders)

The Move: Taking a light dumbbell in each hand, stand with your knees slightly bent and one foot ahead of the other. Bend forward slightly and make sure you keep your heels flat on the floor. Bend your elbows and in slow motion, swing one arm forward and the other back. One up-and-back movement is a rep.

Sets: 4 sets of 25.

The Sly Report: Pretend you're Carl Lewis running the hundred-yard dash in super slo-mo. Bent-over runners build unbelievable rear deltoids and caps. They're also excellent for your glutes and thighs. Beware: your arms will be on fire!

TIP
Try not to be overly rigid on the pull-down, since it can injure your back. It's best to follow your body's natural responses to this move.

65

★ SMITH MACHINE ★ SHOULDER PRESS
(shoulders)

The Move: Standing at a Smith Machine, take hold of a barbell with an overhand grip and rest the bar across your upper chest. Inhale and press the bar straight up. Exhale and slowly bring it back down.

Sets: 2 sets of 10.

The Sly Report: This is one of those dependable moves I've been doing for 35 years or more. It was essential for building my upper chest and deltoids in the Rambo movies.

TIP

As with so many gym exercises, the real work happens in lowering the weight rather than in pushing up. Push up with great enthusiasm but come down twice as slow. Just be careful not to put undue stress on the spine. If you're concerned about your back, try the seated shoulder press.

★ SEATED LATERAL RAISES ★
(shoulders)

The Move: Sit at the edge of a flat bench with a dumbbell in each hand. Leaning forward at a 45-degree-angle, touch the dumbbells under your knees. With your elbows slightly bent, raise the dumbbells with gusto to shoulder level. Slowly return them to the starting position, quietly clinking the dumbbells beneath you. At the very top, you should feel as though you're pouring water out of each dumbbell. The overall effect should be: come up, pour, come up, pour.

Sets: 1 set of 10.

The Sly Report: Another staple of mine, this one isolates the rear part of the deltoids. A must.

TIP
The key is to remain bent over throughout the exercise. The tendency is to want to pop up. Also, control the weights on the way down rather than just dropping them.

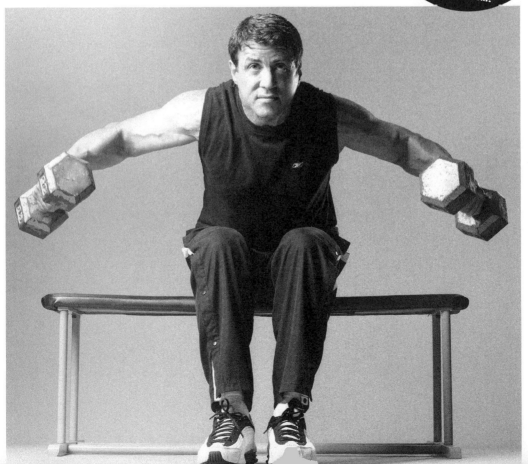

★ PUNCHING DUMBBELLS ★
(shoulders)

The Move: Holding a light (5-pound) dumbbell in each hand, stand in a comfortable position with one knee slightly forward and both knees slightly bent. Punch one arm straight out and bring it back, then punch the other arm out and bring it back. Your hands should twist at the end of the punch (the dumbbells go vertical to horizontal).

Sets: 1 set of 20.

The Sly Report: This move works almost every muscle in your body, especially if you rotate your hands as you punch and twist. You'll see me punching dumbbells at the start of my workouts. It has radically changed my shoulder shape, upper back, and forearms.

TIP
Use a dumbbell weight that is light enough for you to do 20 reps. Don't forget to lean forward with one leg. To add some thrills, try alternating legs with each punch.

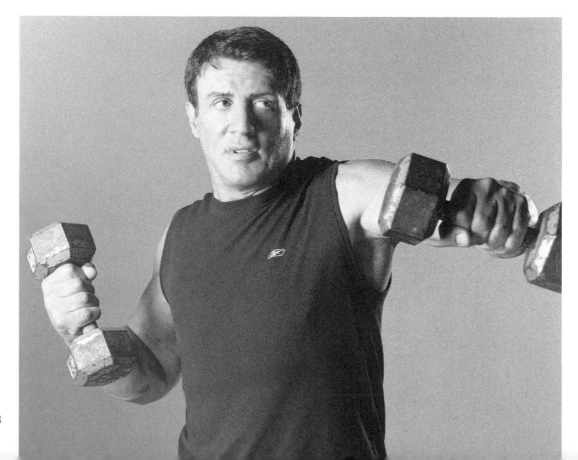

★ BARBELL CURLS ★
(biceps)

The Move: Standing with your feet comfortably apart, take hold of the barbell with palms facing forward and hands at shoulder width. Without leaning back, lift the weight toward you with gusto, exhaling as you go. Pause for a split second at the top and slowly lower the bar until your arms are fully extended, inhaling all the way.

Sets: 3 sets of 8 maximum.

The Sly Report: Nothing makes you feel stronger than biceps strength, and nothing builds biceps like standing barbell curls. It's as honest an exercise as you can find. You can't cheat because it's just you and the barbell. I love this move because there's no wasted effort.

TIP
This move is almost foolproof for building biceps. Just keep your back against the bench and release the weights slowly on the decline.

★ INCLINE DUMBBELL CURLS ★
(biceps)

The Move: Sit on an incline bench, holding a dumbbell in each hand with an underhand grip. With your chest up and back flat against the bench, curl both dumbbells (one at a time or both together) to your shoulders, inhaling on the way up. Then slowly lower the weights on the exhale until your arms are fully extended at your sides.

Sets: 3 sets of 8 maximum.

The Sly Report: Have you ever talked to your muscles? As you bring up the dumbbells, say, "Grow." It's what I call "body dialogue," where I actually converse with certain parts of my body. It keeps me focused on the job at hand rather than daydream, which can happen a lot at the gym. I'll be in the middle of an intense curl and start thinking about something else, and my strength literally drops 50 percent. The gym is a mind game; it's about staying mentally focused. I say talk your way through it!

★ PREACHER CURLS ★
(biceps)

The Move: Sit with your chest against the preacher curl bench, making sure your armpits hug the top of the bench. Take hold of a barbell and extend your arms fully toward the floor. Inhale as you curl the bar up with power toward your biceps. Hold the weights at the top a moment, then slowly lower the bar on the exhale until your arms are once again fully extended.

Sets: 3 sets of 8 maximum.

The Sly Report: If I had to choose one arm exercise, this would be it. Preacher curls add enormous width to the biceps and the position requires you to be incredibly strict. As you'll discover, there's no opportunity for cheating and therefore no wasted effort.

TIP

Preacher curls are all about sculpting the biceps. Watch yourself in the mirror. It will help your form and intensity.

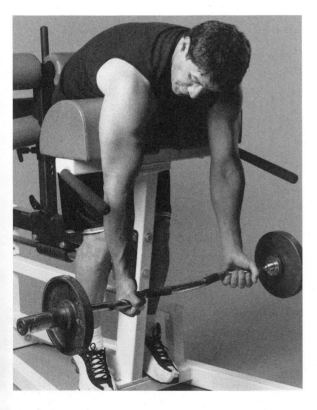
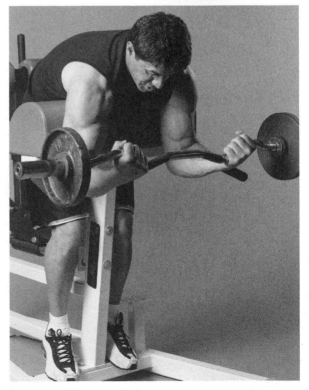

★ LOW PULLEY CURLS ★
(biceps)

The Move: Stand facing the machine and grasp a bar on a low cable pulley with an underhand grip. Keeping your back straight, inhale and curl the pulley toward the biceps. Pause momentarily at the top of the exercise before slowly lowering the pulley to the starting position as you breathe out.

Sets: 3 sets of 10.

The Sly Report: I love this move because it keeps consistent pressure on the biceps all the way up and all the way down. Just a nice, clean exercise.

TIP
For variety, try one-handed low-pulley curls as well as two-arm curls with separate cables.

★ OVERHEAD ROPE ★ PUSH-DOWNS
(triceps)

The Move: Attach a rope extension to the overhead cable and stand facing away from the machine. Lean forward slightly and place one foot slightly ahead of the other. Inhale and push the rope down until your arms are fully extended. It should feel as though you're banging on a huge door with both your fists. Exhale as you slowly raise the rope and lower the weights to the starting position.

Sets: 3 sets of 8.

The Sly Report: This world-class triceps move is really just a variation on cable press-downs. Because the rope is flexible, it allows for a bend in the wrists, which increases the demands on the triceps more than with a straight bar.

TIP
At the end of the release, be mindful not to let the rope go back too far over your head or you'll strain your shoulder joints.

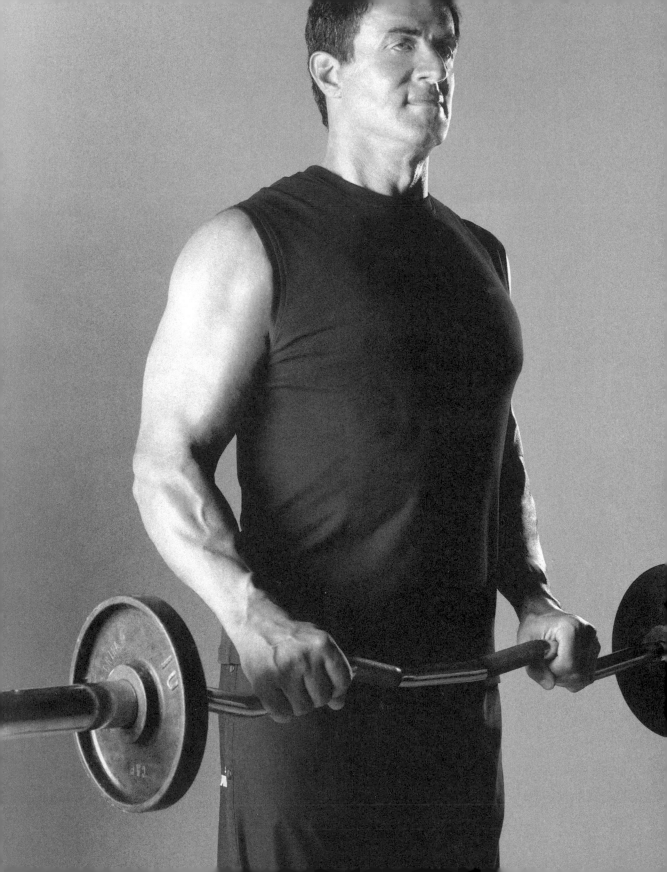

★ BENT-BAR EXTENSIONS ★
(triceps)

The Move: Standing or sitting, take hold of a barbell with a bent bar using an overhand grip. Slowly bring the bar to your chest and lower it to your thighs. Repeat.

Sets: 2 sets of 8 maximum.

The Sly Report: I can always tell if a guy's in shape by the shape of his triceps. Practically speaking, you can only develop triceps in the gym, so it's a sign that somebody is working out and tending to his body.

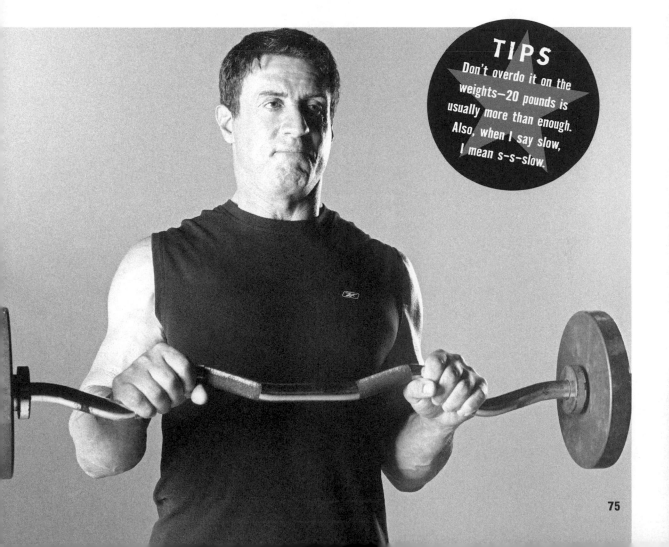

TIPS
Don't overdo it on the weights—20 pounds is usually more than enough. Also, when I say slow, I mean s-s-slow.

★ CABLE PRESS-DOWNS ★
(triceps)

The Move: Attach a short or bent bar to the overhead cable and stand facing the machine. Lean forward slightly but keep your elbows tight against your body. Inhale and push the bar down until your arms are fully extended. Exhale as you slowly release the bar and lower the weights to the starting position, keeping your elbows against your body the whole way.

Sets: 4 sets of 12.

The Sly Report: A gym classic. Press-downs are great for beginners because they help develop strength for more difficult exercises. Serious athletes love what they do for the back of the arms.

TIP
This move has many variations. You can use a long bar and take a wider grip or you can use a rope. You can face away from the machine or do it on your knees. Bodybuilders sometimes do one-handed press-downs.

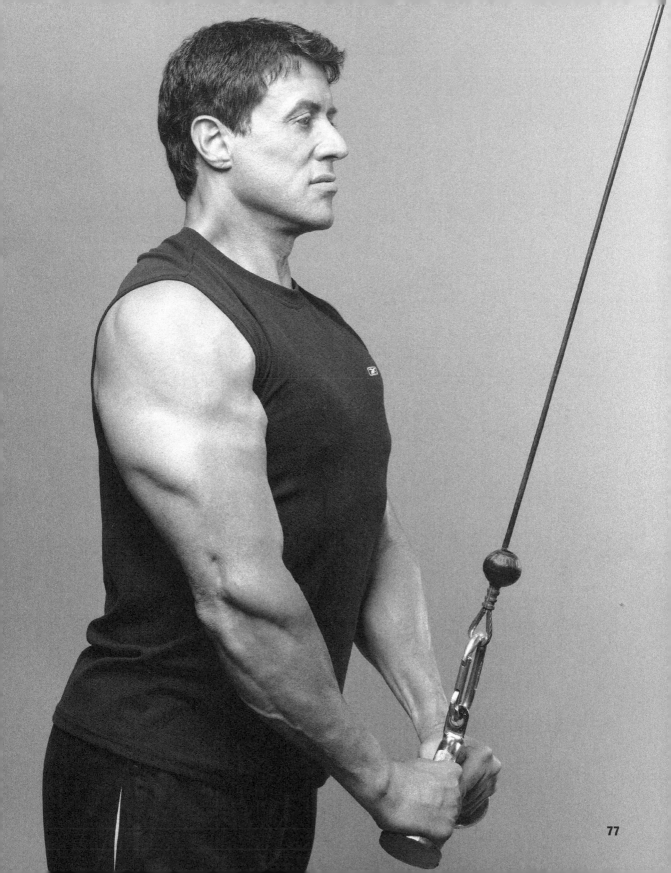

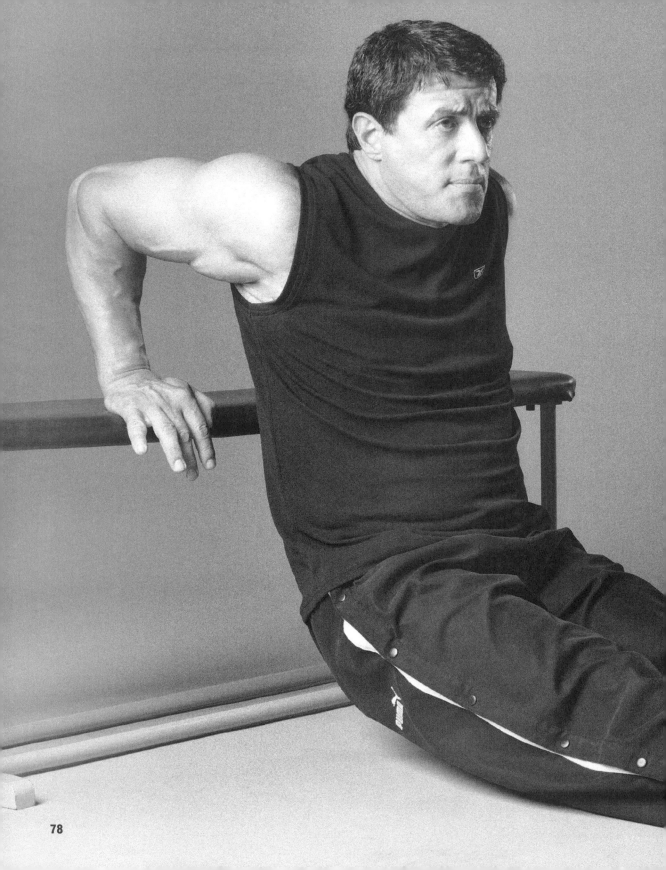

★ TRICEPS DIPS ★
(triceps)

The Move: Put the heels of your hands on the edge of a flat bench behind you at shoulder width. Keeping your hands on the bench, take a breath as you press yourself up until your elbows are locked. Keep your legs at either a 45-degree angle to the floor or fully extend them. Exhale and slowly lower yourself almost to the floor.

Sets: 3 sets of 10.

The Sly Report: Some people like doing these at the dip station, but I prefer the bench because it gives you a fuller range of motion. Plus, you can do it almost anywhere.

TIP

When people do this wrong, they usually don't go down far enough. You should feel your clothes touching the ground at the bottom of the dip, otherwise you're not engaging the heads of the triceps. If you want to increase the intensity, rest your feet on a parallel bench and do the exercise with a barbell weight in your lap.

★ REVERSE WRIST CURLS ★
(forearms)

The Move: Grab a bar with an overhand grip and sit on a flat bench with the bar resting comfortably on your lap, just above your knees. Without lifting your hands, curl the weight up by flexing your wrists in a strong upward motion. Slowly lower the bar and repeat.

Sets: 2 sets of 8 maximum.

The Sly Report: This is a great exercise for developing powerful forearms, which to me are real indicators of strength and conditioning. Reverse curls also build up the grip, which tends to weaken as we get older.

TIP
No need to set any records on this one. Use a light weight.

★ HAMMER CURLS ★
(forearms)

The Move: Stand with a dumbbell in each hand, palms facing inward. Extend your arms so they are hanging straight down by your sides. Inhale and curl the weights toward your shoulders, either together or one at a time. The hard part: *Slowly* lower the dumbbells until your arms are fully extended again. Remember to breathe out as you bring the weights down.

Sets: 3 sets of 8 maximum.

The Sly Report: The hammer curl is an exercise I learned from a fellow named Carl Weathers, an actor better known as Apollo Creed, Rocky's nemesis. It's an interesting exercise that accentuates the tops of the forearms, which are grossly neglected. Specifically, the move builds the brachialis and brachioradialis, which are the muscles above and below the elbow. Men can get strong quickly using this technique, and if done consistently, it will create an explosion of strength in any endeavor that requires hand power, such as tennis or golf. Thanks, Carl!

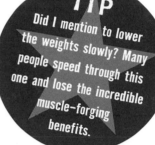

TIP
Did I mention to lower the weights slowly? Many people speed through this one and lose the incredible muscle-forging benefits.

★ FLAT BENCH WRIST CURLS ★
(forearms)

The Move: Sitting on a flat bench, take an underhand grip on a set of dumbbells and rest your wrists on your knees. Inhale and curl the weights up and take the weights as far as you can. Exhale and slowly return the dumbbells to the starting position.

Sets: 2 sets of 10 maximum.

The Sly Report: It's one of the best hand and forearm exercises, but watching someone doing wrist curls, you'd swear they weren't doing anything. Trust me, that little upward flick of the wrist is a major challenge. In fact, you shouldn't be able to do more than 8 or 10 reps without feeling an intense burn. I like this exercise because it really affects your everyday life. Rolling the wrist back and forth brings a great deal of blood flow and flexibility to the metacarpals (the flexor muscles of the wrists) and keeps the hands and fingers feeling vital and energized. That's incredibly helpful if you use computers, play sports, or do anything else with your hands.

TIP
You can also do this move with a barbell or on the gym's wrist-curl machine.

★ HANGS ★
(forearms)

The Move: Grab hold of a high bar with an overhand grip, your hands wider than shoulder width apart. Keeping a slight bend in the elbows, hang from the bar. You should feel an intense burn in your arms.

Sets: Build up to 30 seconds if you dare.

The Sly Report: Who says you can't get in great shape just hanging around the gym? This is something I started doing with Dolph Lundgren in *Rocky IV* because it gives a huge pump to your forearm and taxes arm and back muscles you would never normally activate. I would estimate that 95 percent of the world can't hold on for more than 45 seconds. When you get up to a minute and a half or two minutes, you're in rare air. Meanwhile, two sets of twenty to 30 seconds will do you just fine.

TIP
The bar must be deep in your palm.

★ WRIST ★ ROLLERS
(forearms)

The Move: Hold a wrist-roller device with your arms completely extended. Rotate one wrist at a time to bring the cable up around the roller. Keep rolling until the weight reaches the top. Then reverse the motion in order to return the weight slowly to the starting position.

Sets: 1 set of 3 up, 3 down.

The Sly Report: This is the most intense forearm exercise going. I used this one a lot for *Cliffhanger*. Wrist rollers are also known to prevent carpal tunnel syndrome.

TIP
To up the ante on rollers, do them with a lighter weight but with your arms locked straight out in front of you.

★ RAMBO PULL-DOWNS ★
(back)

The Move: Using an overhand grip, grab the ends of a wide bar on a cable pull-down machine and sit with your knees secured snugly under the support pads. Pull the bar to the top (rather than the center) of your chest, keeping your elbows directly below the bar. Slowly return the bar back to the starting position. Breathe in as you pull the bar down; breathe out on the slow release.

Sets: 2 sets of 10 maximum.

The Sly Report: Wide-grip lat pull-downs are the shortest route between you and an expansive, V-shaped back. For *Rambo III*, I committed myself to developing a very wide back. I remember when the movie came out, there was a gigantic billboard on Sunset Boulevard. I was facing away from the camera and the billboard simply read, RAMBO'S BACK. So this exercise really paid off. The wide-grip pull-down was one of my mainstays then and continues to be. It's a gravity-defeating move in that it lifts all the muscles of the back, particularly the lower ones, which tend to sag without use.

TIP If the extremely wide grip isn't comfortable, bring your hands in a little. Your hands should be slightly wider than your shoulders. Also, don't lean too far back when you're bringing down the weights. Beginners like this machine because it builds strength for doing chin-ups.

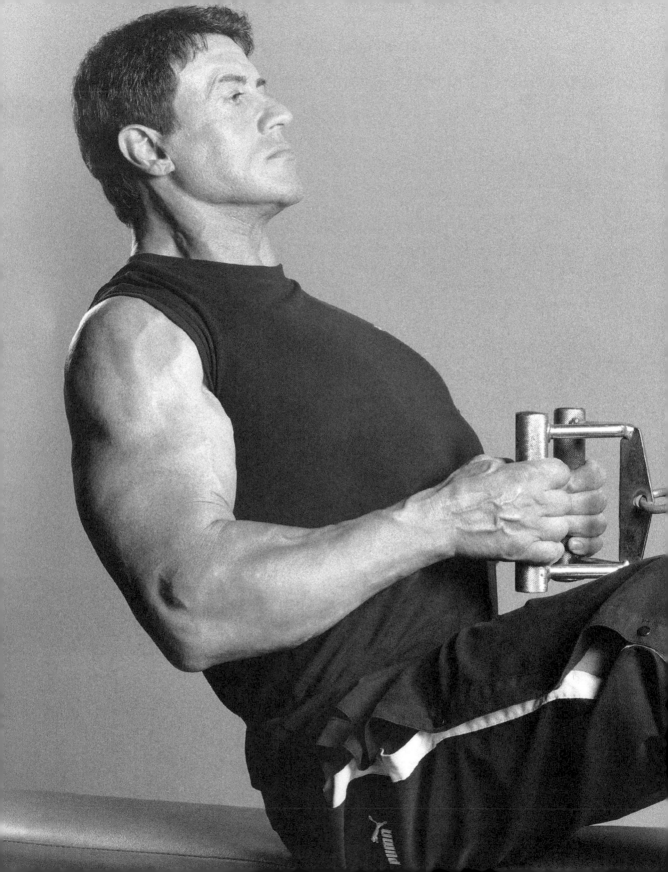

★ SEATED ROWS ★
(back)

The Move: As you're seated facing the machine, bend your knees and secure your feet on the foot plate. Lean forward and grab hold of the pulley handle. Take a breath and pull the handle until your body returns to the seated upright position. Slowly return the weights to the starting position, exhaling as you complete the move. To avoid back injuries, keep your spine relatively straight. Never round your back.

Sets: 2 sets of 10 maximum.

The Sly Report: This is a fun move that focuses primarily on the latissimus dorsi in the center of the back, the largest muscle in the body. It's also excellent for the biceps, forearms, shoulders, lower back, quads, and hamstrings.

TIP
Be sure to complete the full range of motion by drawing the handle until your shoulders are back and spine is straight, then releasing the weights all the way to the starting position.

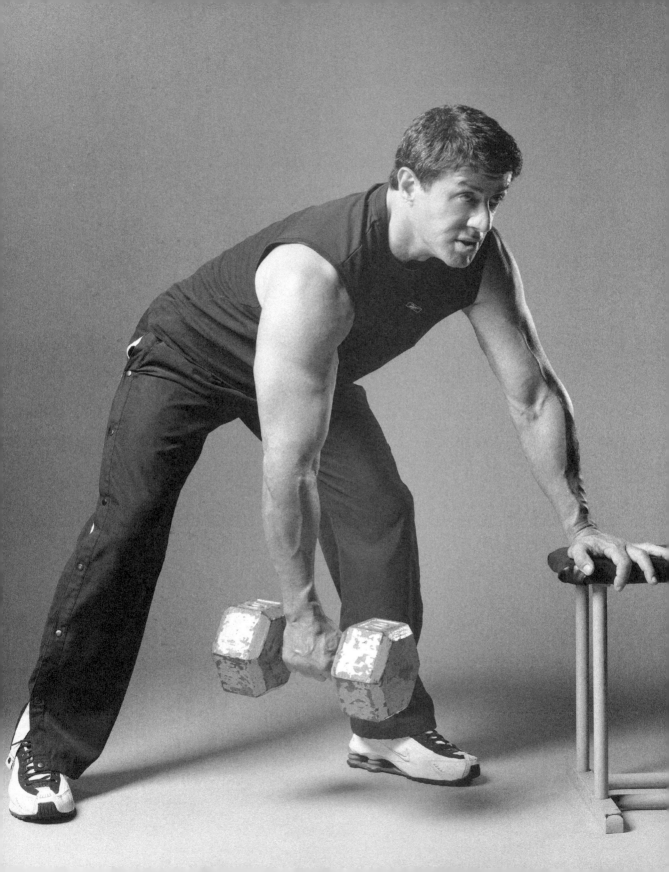

★ ONE-ARM DUMBBELL ROWS ★
(back)

The Move: Stand with a dumbbell in one hand and with the other hand holding a flat bench for support. Lower the dumbbell so the arm hangs straight down. Leaning forward slightly, raise the dumbbell by drawing your elbow back in a forceful move. Slowly lower the weight until your arm is fully extended.

Sets: 2 sets of 8 maximum.

The Sly Report: This one's a bit more difficult, but it's absolutely worth the effort. The act of pulling up builds your back and neck muscles as well as your biceps and grip. It's not a very popular exercise, but if you're serious about changing your body structure, this will work like nothing else.

TIP
You can also do this with one leg bent at the knee resting flat on the bench.

★ DUMBBELL SHRUGS ★
(back)

The Move: Stand with your feet comfortably apart and a dumbbell in each hand, arms extended at your sides. Inhale as you raise your shoulders to your ears without bending your arms, as if you were hoisting two heavy suitcases. Slowly lower to the starting position, exhaling along the way. As you do the shrugs, say to yourself, "I don't know, I don't know, I don't know."

Sets: 2 sets of 8 maximum.

The Sly Report: A lot of guys do not do shrugs and that's a mistake. We don't do enough lifting in our daily lives to fortify the trapezoid muscles at the base of the neck, and they tend to atrophy. We need strong trapezoids to hold the shoulders up and support the upper back, especially as we age. That's why maintaining the trapezius is vital. It's also just a great-looking muscle when it's properly developed. If you look at Greek sculptures or Michelangelo's *David*, you'll notice a beautiful curved line, almost like a small mountain ridge, connecting the neck to the arms. *That's* the trapezius.

TIP
At the top of the shrug, squeeze and hold for a count of 2.

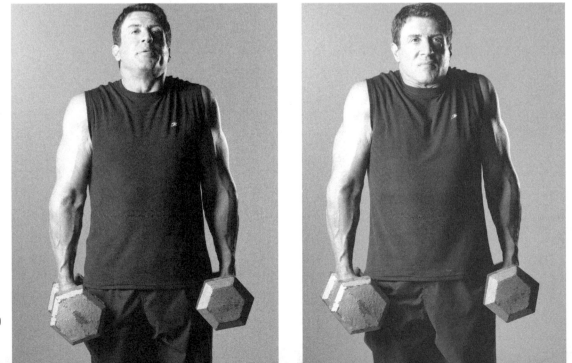

★ HYPEREXTENSIONS ★
(back and buttocks)

The Move: Lie facedown on a hyperextension or back-extension bench, securing your ankles under the ankle supports. Your upper thighs should lie flat across the main padding, leaving enough room for you to bend forward at the waist. Hold your hands behind your head or in front of you, or cross your arms at your chest. Slowly bend forward at the waist as far as you can while keeping your back flat. Then raise your upper body until your legs and torso are in a straight line again (arching up further can injure your back). Breathe out while you lower your torso and breathe in as you raise it.

Sets: 2 sets of 8 maximum.

The Sly Report: The hyperextension is an extraordinary exercise that ranks among the best exercises out there for the glutes and lower back. It's worked wonders for me, and I've seen it deliver extraordinary results for many boxers.

TIP
If you have a bad back, this is going to get rid of it if you start slowly and gently.

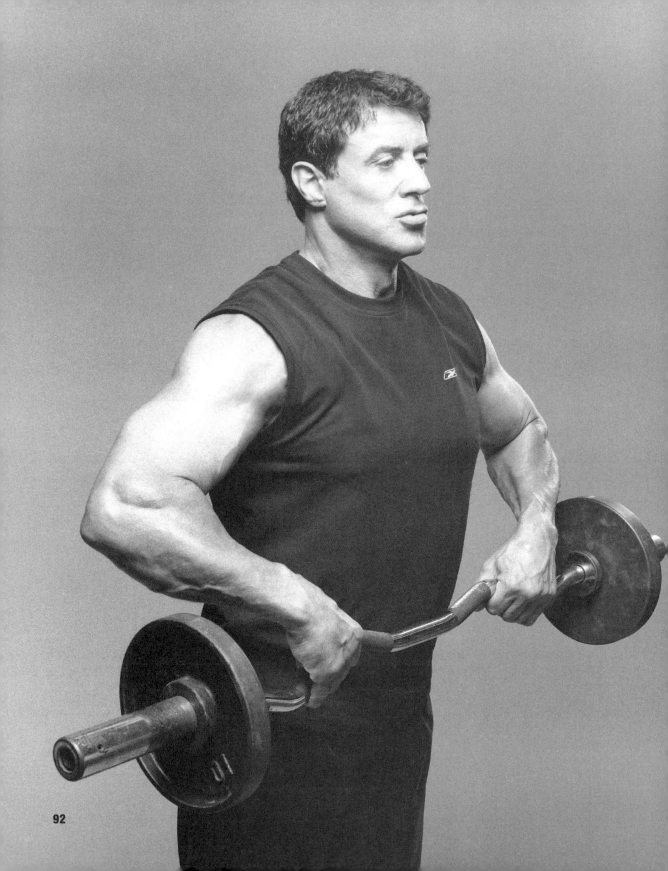

★ UPRIGHT ROWS ★
(back)

The Move: Take an overhand grip on a barbell and stand with your feet slightly apart and back straight. You'll want to have a medium to wide grip on the bar. On the inhale, pull the bar straight up until it touches your chin, bringing your elbows up and out. It should feel like you've been caught naked and are pulling the sheet up quickly to cover yourself. Exhale and slowly lower the barbell to the starting position.

Sets: 4 sets of 10.

The Sly Report: What an intense workout for the trapezius! Feel free to use a straight barbell, but I like the bent bar because it focuses intensity on the forearm flexors and doesn't hurt the wrist as much.

TIP
The wider the grip, the more you work the deltoid muscles. Use a shorter grip to attack the trapezius.

★ ROCKY CHINS ★
(back)

The Move: Take a wide overhand grip on a high chin-up bar. Inhale and pull yourself up until you're eye-to-eye with the bar. Here's the hard part: *Slowly* lower yourself to the starting position as you exhale. Then do another one.

Sets: Work your way up to 20 or more reps.

The Sly Report: Chins are the forgotten exercise. With the arms wide, you address the muscles of the central back: the trapezius, lats, and rhomboideus in particular. Of course, your arms also get a massive workout. I like any exercise where you're working with your own body weight.

TIP

I often do these with my palms facing inward so I can strengthen my biceps and lats.

94

★ NARROW-GRIP PULL-DOWNS ★
(back)

The Move: Keeping your hands close together, take an underhand grip on an overhead cable bar and sit facing the machine with your knees secured snugly under the support pads. Inhale as you pull the bar to the top (rather than the center) of your chest, arching your back slightly. Slowly return the bar to the starting position as you breathe out.

Sets: 2 sets of 10 maximum.

The Sly Report: I think the narrow-grip pull-downs are more important than the wide-grip for overall strength. This move builds the center of the back—the upper trapezius—and brings the shoulder blades closer together, so the back radiates power and makes you feel more forceful. To understand what you're dealing with, draw an imaginary bow. Those are the muscles we're targeting here. The wide grip does incredible things cosmetically in terms of building that desirable *V*. But when you look at a man from behind, if his back is wide, you know he's not nearly as strong as the man whose back is thick. And nothing builds thick musculature like this.

TIP

Try not to be overly rigid on the pull-down, since it can injure your back. It's best to follow your body's natural responses to this move.

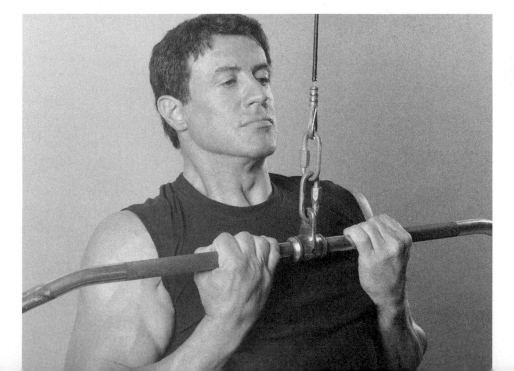

★ SMITH MACHINE HALF-SQUATS ★
(legs)

The Move: At the Smith Machine, stand straight with a barbell across your shoulders behind your neck. Using a fairly wide overhand grip, slowly lower your hips until your thighs are parallel with the floor. You should almost feel like you're sitting on a chair. Once you're at the bottom, press back up with power to a standing position, looking straight ahead and keeping your spine erect. Take a deep breath on the way down and exhale as you thrust back up.

Sets: 2 sets of 10.

The Sly Report: Squats are probably my least favorite exercise in the gym, but they're essential for building strong legs. Half-squats are all you need to firm up the quadriceps so be sure not to dip too deeply on the downward side of this move. I've had more than my share of problems overdoing it with squats (see box).

TIP

If you can stand on your toes on the way up, it's a freebie for the calves. Squeeze your butt every time you push up. By the way, you can do this move with or without a Smith Machine. I like using it because you don't have to balance the weight on your shoulder and therefore can focus exclusively on the task at hand.

TO SQUAT OR NOT TO SQUAT?

Squats are the most powerful exercises for the legs ever created. I recommend you only do controlled half-squats when first starting out.

I went to extremes training for the film *Cliffhanger*. That's when I had the biggest legs of my career. In those days, I was doing squats split-legged, where one leg would go out in front of the other. Then I'd do wide squats. I even tried one-legged squats in the Smith Machine. They wreaked havoc on my knees. Are squats necessary to have strong, shapely legs? Not really. It's a matter of choice. You can get wonderful results doing leg exercises that are not so difficult.

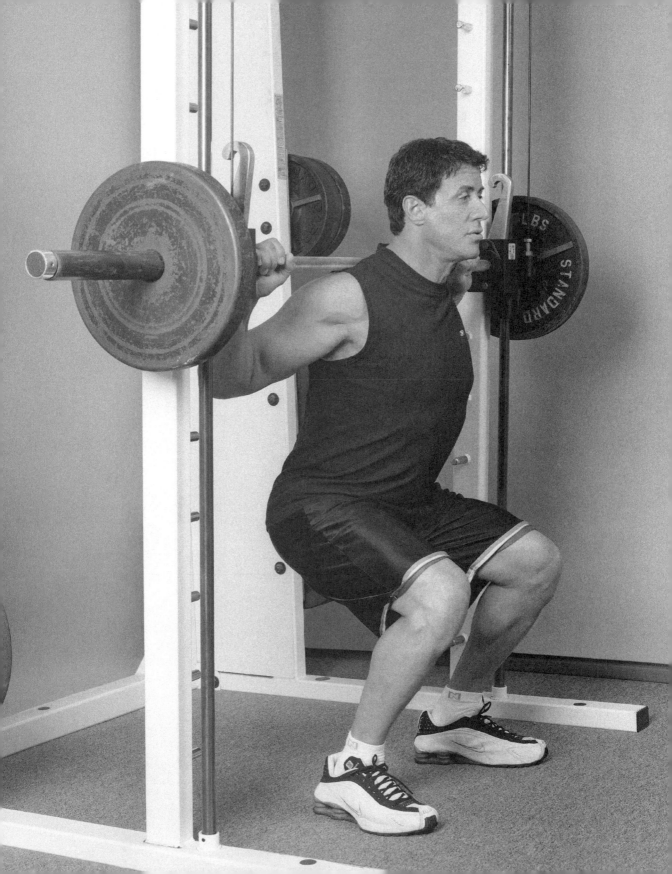

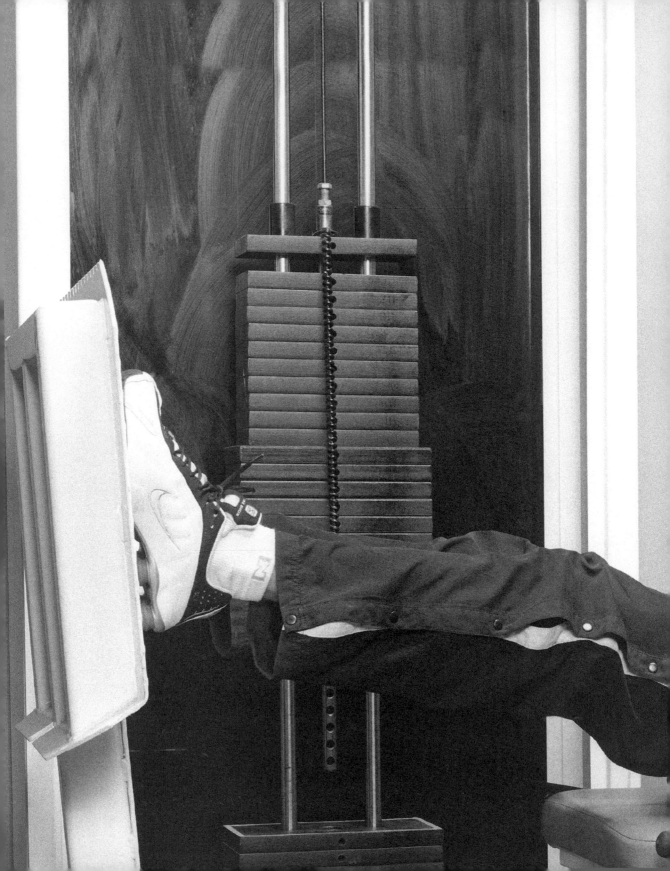

★ LEG PRESSES ★
(legs)

The Move: Lie back in the leg-press machine with your feet firmly on the platform, slightly wider than shoulder-width apart. Extend your legs to release the stoppers but maintain a slight bend in the knees. Exhale as you slowly draw your knees back, lowering the platform and weights.

Sets: 2 sets of 10.

The Sly Report: This one looks so comfortable. Lie down and good night, right? Not exactly. The leg press delivers a hard-core assault on the quadriceps, hamstrings, and glutes. In fact, it works just about every muscle in the body. Leg presses are especially good for building the power and thickness of the front thighs.

TIP
Don't lock your knees at the top of the exercise. It puts too much stress on the joints.

★ LEG EXTENSIONS ★
(legs)

The Move: Sit back at the leg extension machine with your ankles tucked securely behind the support pads. Inhale as you power up with your legs. Contract your quads at the top of the motion. Slowly return the weights to the starting position with a long breath out.

Sets: 2 sets of 10.

The Sly Report: This is another deceptively comfortable-looking exercise, but leg extensions definitely aren't for La-Z-Boy types. This one hammers the quadriceps and hip flexors and creates gladiator thighs. Although it's not my favorite exercise, I do it because it secures the knee in place, which serves you well if you enjoy jogging or simply endeavor to feel more security and spring in your normal gait.

TIP

As you do this move, tighten your abs as a bonus prize for your gut.

★ LYING LEG CURLS ★
(legs)

The Move: Lie facedown on a leg-curl machine with your lower legs secured under the roller pads. Grab the handles and take a breath as you raise your feet upward. Draw your heels as close to your buttocks as possible. Exhale as you slowly return your legs to the starting position.

Sets: 3 sets of 10.

The Sly Report: This is an exercise I truly hate, but it's a necessary evil. It attacks the hamstrings, which are so important for feeling athletic. It also builds up the buttocks. It's important not to overuse this exercise. I've seen a lot of bodybuilders focus so much on it that they literally build hamstrings that look like softballs and they end up with a jerky gait. But as part of a balanced regimen, it's a good addition for overall strength and dexterity.

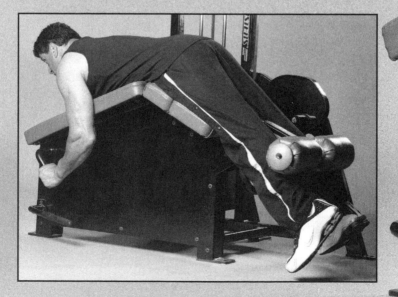

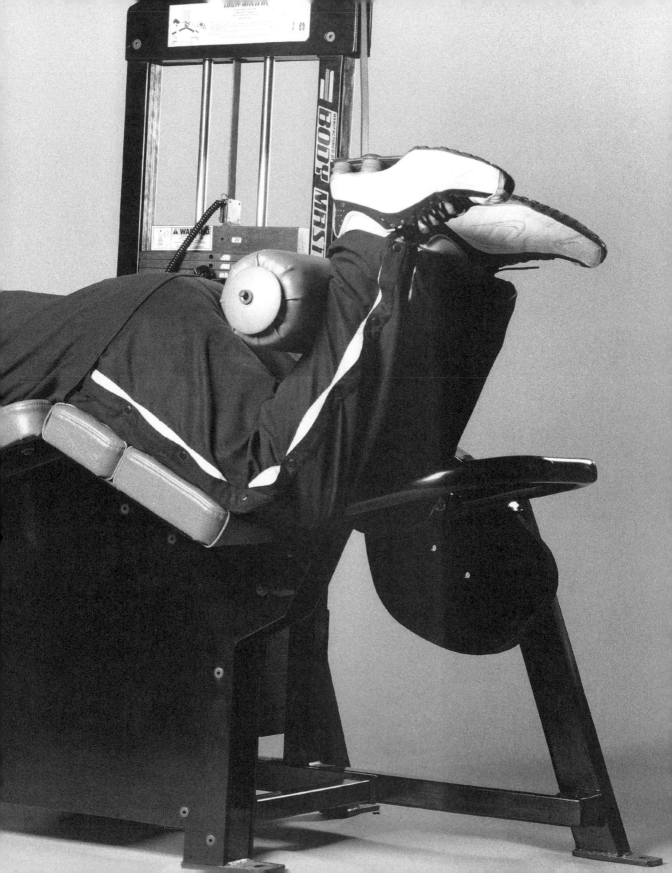

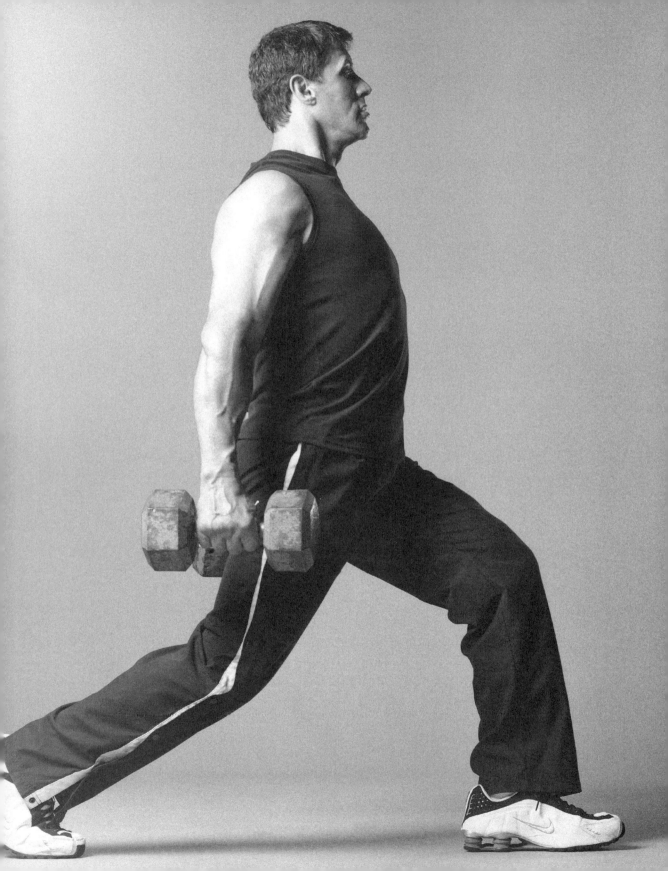

★ HALF-LUNGES ★
(legs and buttocks)

The Move: Keeping your body ramrod straight, take a step forward so that your front knee forms a right angle to the floor. Your forward knee must not extend beyond your toes. Your back leg should be elongated with the knee remaining a few inches off the ground. Step back to the starting position and repeat the exercise, stepping forward with the other leg. You can do this move with or without dumbbells in your hands.

Sets: 2 sets of 8 to 10.

The Sly Report: It may sound funny, but a strong butt helps put power in your step. When your butt is solid, you're creating a good foundation that helps your posture, your gait, and your balance. It also makes you feel immovable, like society is not about to push you out of the way.

TIP
The front foot must remain flat against the floor even though you may be tempted to raise your heel. If you're on your toes, you are stepping too far forward.

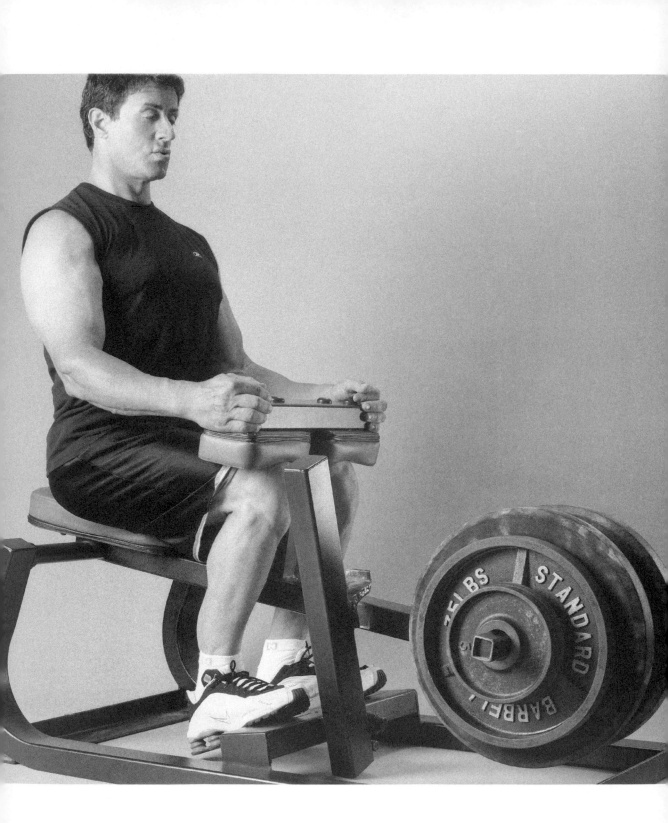

★ SEATED CALF RAISES ★
(calves)

The Move: Seated at the calf machine, secure your knees snugly under the support pads and place the balls of your feet on the footrest. Grip the knee rest and slowly lower your heels as far as possible, then press back up on your toes until your calves are fully contracted. Repeat with a slow, steady rhythm.

Sets: 2 sets of 8 maximum.

TIP
Keep your back straight and avoid rocking your body and using momentum to lift the weight.

The Sly Report: Making a real difference with your calves is tough. If you intend to build them up and add inches, it will take an inordinate amount of work. But if you're just looking to keep them in shape, this is a fine exercise. I see this as an optional exercise, because you tone your calves naturally doing other exercises such as riding the stationary bike and walking.

★ CARDIO FINALE ★

The Move: Split this exercise between two cardio machines of your choice to get your heart rate up between 130 and 150 beats per minute. Rowing machines are the best. Build to an intensity level of 8 or 9 out of 10.

Time: 15 minutes split between two cardio machines.

The Sly Report: You've had a strong workout. Now it's time to energize with a cardio finale. Like I said, I've basically planned my vacations to avoid aerobic conditioning and didn't really do it at all until I got into the ring for the original *Rocky*. The trouble is, if you don't get the heart pumping, you don't build lung power or stamina. The key for me is trying new machines, like the VersaClimber or a rowing machine, which make you sweat like nobody's business.

TIP
Go hard enough to feel strain but no pain.

THE DRILLS

Here are my day-to-day guides for working out. If you're new to weight training or not feeling as powerful as you'd like, start with the Classic Workout for Mondays, Wednesdays, and Fridays. After you're jamming on the Classics, you'll want to push to the next level, the Advanced Workout, which is also three days a week. In both the Classic and Advanced Workouts, the Friday drills are the same as Monday's. Then, when you're ready for the ultimate challenge, take a crack at SuperSets. I've also included a workout tailor-made for women, though women can certainly benefit from any of these moves.

There's absolutely no need to rush to advanced levels. We're talking about a lifetime commitment here. I'd much rather you take it slow and enjoy the process than risk burning out too quickly. And remember, mistakes are okay. It's the way we know we're challenging ourselves.

Finally, a note about time. In the beginning, it will take a while to get these moves down, so expect to spend at least two hours at the gym each visit. Once you get the hang of things, you won't spend more than an hour and a half each day. There's more to life than being at the gym.

CLASSIC Workout

Monday and Friday Drills

1. Cardio Warm-up
2. Floor Crunches (abdominals)
3. Hanging Raises (abdominals)
4. Incline Bench Press (chest)
5. Wide-Arm Push-ups (chest)
6. Smith Machine Shoulder Press (shoulders)
7. Seated Lateral Raises (shoulders)
8. Punching Dumbbells (shoulders)
9. Incline Bench Dumbbell Flys (chest)
10. Bent-Bar Extensions (triceps)
11. Half-Lunges (legs and buttocks)
12. Extra Credit: Seated Calf Raises (calves)
13. Cardio Finale

Wednesday Drills

1. Cardio Warm-up
2. Twisting Crunches (abdominals)
3. Barbell Curls (biceps)
4. Incline Dumbbell Curls (biceps)
5. Reverse Wrist Curls (forearms)
6. Rambo Pull-downs (back)
7. Seated Rows (back)
8. One-Arm Dumbbell Rows (back)
9. Dumbbell Shrugs (back)
10. Hyperextensions (back)
11. Cardio Finale

ADVANCED Workout

Monday and Friday Drills

1. Cardio Warm-up
2. Hanging Raises (abdominals)
3. Twisting Crunches (abdominals)
4. Incline Bench Dumbbell Flys (chest)
5. Wide-Arm Push-ups (chest)
6. Rambo Pull-downs (back)
7. One-Arm Dumbbell Rows (back)
8. Dumbbell Shrugs (back)
9. Smith Machine Half Squats (legs)
10. Leg Presses (legs)
11. Leg Extensions (legs)
12. Cardio Finale

Wednesday Drills

1. Cardio Warm-up
2. Smith Machine Shoulder Press (shoulders)
3. Bent-Over Runners (shoulders)
4. Upright Rows (back)
5. Dumbbell Shrugs (back)
6. Rocky Chins (back)
7. Barbell Curls (biceps)
8. Cable Press-downs (triceps)
9. Overhead Rope Push-downs (Triceps)
10. Triceps Dips (triceps)
11. Flat Bench Wrist Curls (forearms)
12. Narrow-Grip Pull-downs (back)
13. Wrist Rollers (forearms)
14. Cardio Finale

SUPERSETS WORKOUT

A SuperSet happens when you move from one exercise directly into another without a break. There should be a seamless transition from one to another for the best results. The idea is to work opposing muscle groups—like triceps and biceps or abs and lower back muscles—in order to really put them to the test.

What's the point? I believe the body can become indifferent to exercise after a while, and sometimes you simply need to recharge the engine. SuperSetting is like taking your car up to 120 miles an hour. It engages a lot of machinery that normally wouldn't be taxed. It causes the brain and every muscle in your body to go on red alert. I think it's a must if you expect to make real progress over time in the gym.

Usually, I'll do SuperSets once every other month for about a week. Then I return to my regular routine with a renewed sense of strength and vigor. It's hard-core, but I think you'll love the results. Here's what to do:

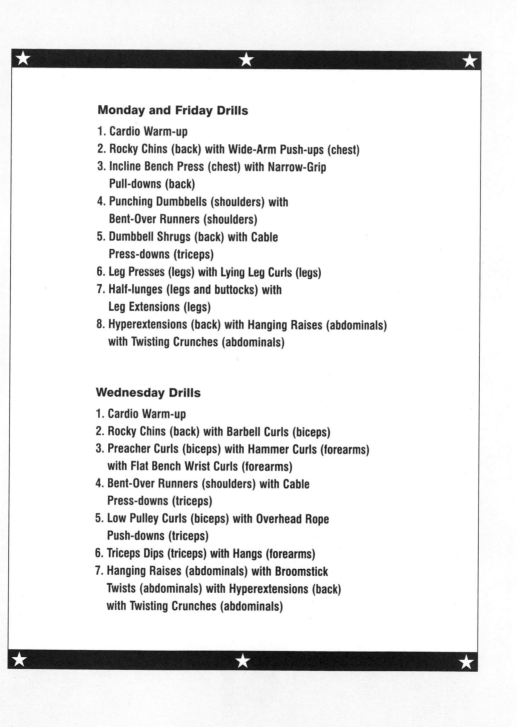

Monday and Friday Drills

1. Cardio Warm-up
2. Rocky Chins (back) with Wide-Arm Push-ups (chest)
3. Incline Bench Press (chest) with Narrow-Grip
   Pull-downs (back)
4. Punching Dumbbells (shoulders) with
   Bent-Over Runners (shoulders)
5. Dumbbell Shrugs (back) with Cable
   Press-downs (triceps)
6. Leg Presses (legs) with Lying Leg Curls (legs)
7. Half-lunges (legs and buttocks) with
   Leg Extensions (legs)
8. Hyperextensions (back) with Hanging Raises (abdominals)
   with Twisting Crunches (abdominals)

Wednesday Drills

1. Cardio Warm-up
2. Rocky Chins (back) with Barbell Curls (biceps)
3. Preacher Curls (biceps) with Hammer Curls (forearms)
   with Flat Bench Wrist Curls (forearms)
4. Bent-Over Runners (shoulders) with Cable
   Press-downs (triceps)
5. Low Pulley Curls (biceps) with Overhead Rope
   Push-downs (triceps)
6. Triceps Dips (triceps) with Hangs (forearms)
7. Hanging Raises (abdominals) with Broomstick
   Twists (abdominals) with Hyperextensions (back)
   with Twisting Crunches (abdominals)

SEVEN WAYS TO ENERGIZE YOUR WORKOUT

1 GO EARLY: It's just easier to feel motivated in the mornings, which is why I get to the gym around 10:45 AM. That's a bit late for some people, but my energy level is still high at that time and I'm not distracted by the commitments of the day. Getting my heart rate up early pretty much guarantees I'll feel positive and vital for the rest of the day. Perhaps that's why the people who exercise most consistently, according to various studies, are the ones who do it early in the morning.

2 DRESS THE PART: You go to the gym to look and feel better. Start with what you're wearing. Wear something that makes you feel athletic or comfortable or sexy or all of the above. It's a sign of respect for what you're doing. I see guys rolling out of bed—celebrities, by the way—wearing these big wrinkled T-shirts, hair all messed up. It's like they're in denial that they're actually at a gym. And guess what? Their workouts are just as uninspired.

3 FUEL UP: Never go to the gym on an empty stomach. You need something in the engine, preferably high-octane fuel. Eating a small piece of fruit and some healthy carbs within 15–30 minutes of exercising elevates the blood sugar level, which helps kick-start the workout. A small bowl of oatmeal with peaches or melon does the trick. So does a banana and a handful of almonds. There are some great energy bars and gels out there, too. Above all, drink water before, during, and after the workout.

4 JAVA, MAN: I believe in slamming back a megadose of coffee before working out. Caffeine helps prime the pump and gives you a natural lift. Many people, myself included, find that it delays fatigue and diminishes the overall sense of exertion, which makes exercise more fun. It also increases alertness, speeds the body's ability to metabolize fat, and stimulates the release of free fatty acids, which are used for energy when you exercise. There are other health benefits, too. In 2004, a Harvard School of

Public Health study found a firm link between coffee and the prevention of Type II, or "adult-onset," diabetes. Men in the study who drank six or more cups a day reduced their diabetes risk by 54 percent.

5 GET THEE TO A TRAINER: Can you do it alone? Yes. Can you do it better with someone else? Absolutely. For the uninitiated, there's a lot of strange equipment in a gym and you need an expert to take you through the paces. Even if it costs a few extra dollars, the guidance will save you medical and chiropractic bills down the road. Not to mention the psychological advantage you'll get. I've been working out for 40 years and I still find myself looking for excuses to slack off in the gym. That's why I need somebody else, somebody who's paid to kick my butt into shape.

6 PLAY THAT FUNKY MUSIC: Just make sure it's something that moves you. Everyone has a music preference and usually it's a generational thing. I like the R&B classics, groups like the Temptations and the Spinners. You can't go wrong with hip-hop, either, whether it's Usher or Nelly or whoever's hot. But if I'm feeling really sluggish, I'll put on something totally out of left field. Once, Jennifer and I were at the gym with Jamie Lee Curtis, Angelina Jolie, Jennifer Connelly, and Christina Applegate and I just threw on some loud bluegrass. They looked at me like I had two heads. Except Jamie Lee, who liked it. The point is, when things get dull, switch up.

7 FOLLOW THE BEAT: Wearing a heart monitor takes your workout to a whole new level. You can see how many calories you're burning, watch your heart rate improve over time, and see where you stand against the standard for your age and weight. Many of the new devices let you download data to your computer, where you can track and analyze your workouts. Plus, they tell you when it's time to go home.

★

THE BOXER'S WORKOUT

From *Rocky* to *The Contender*, training with boxers over the years has taught me so much about staying lean and mean. Here are some of my favorite boxing fitness tricks. Feel free to add them to your regular routine.

1. Skipping: Great boxers are usually great skippers. You probably haven't thought about skipping since third grade, but it's actually an incredibly athletic move and much harder than running. Try it. When I was training for the *Rocky* movies, I'd try skipping a quarter mile and I was usually gasping the whole way.

2. Tiptoes: Stand on your tiptoes for 10 seconds, then start to lower and lift, lower and lift. Do it 10 times and repeat for two sets. It builds your calves and develops unshakeable balance.

3. Water Punches: One of my favorite photographs is a shot of Muhammad Ali training in a pool. He's underwater throwing punches and you can just tell he's bursting with strength. I used the same move training for the *Rocky* films. Water provides great resistance and alleviates the pressure on the joints.

4. Ankle Weights: Strapping two to five pounds around each ankle is one of the best ways to maximize your regular workout. The extra weight gives you an extraordinary workout and you burn fat and build muscle much faster. And when you take those weights off, you feel like you're flying free for the rest of the day.

5. Driving Spikes: My brother, Frank, is an amateur historian of boxing and he's uncovered all kinds of fascinating old-school training techniques that I put to use in my movies. In the old days, many boxers didn't have gyms, so they'd lift rocks, haul water, chop trees, and chase chickens, like I did in *Rocky II*. Pounding spikes into the ground with a big sledgehammer is another great move for building speed and coordination and just blowing off steam. Not recommended, however, unless you don't mind smashing your foot by mistake.

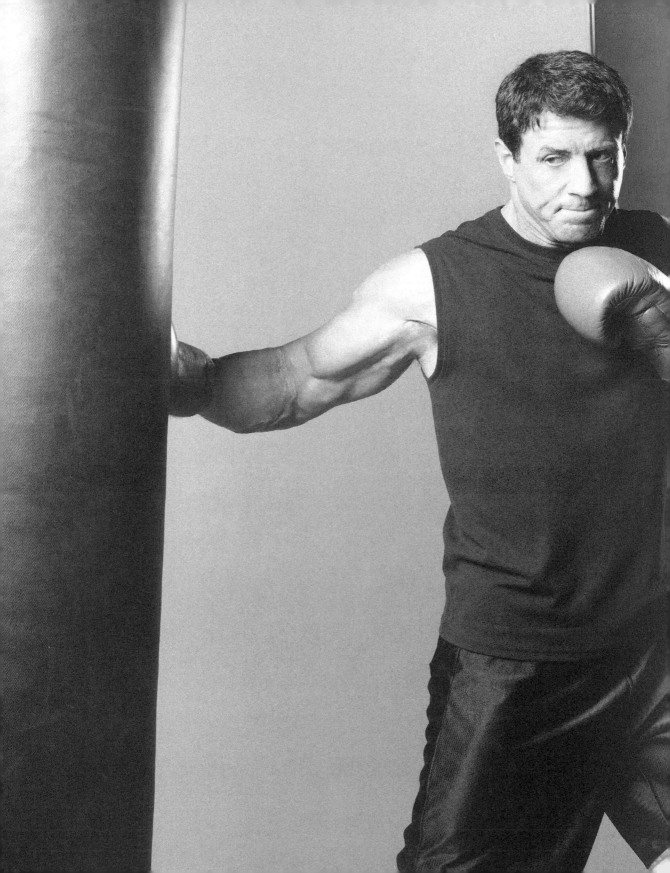

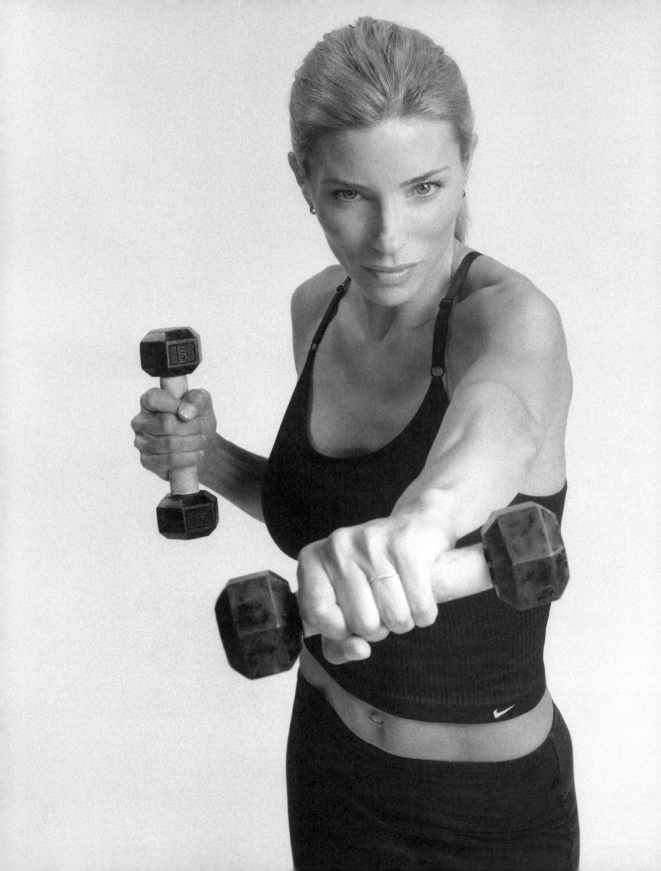

SLY MOVES FOR WOMEN

Most women I know are reluctant to try weight training. Even the athletic types who spend an hour pounding the StairMaster or who'll jog five miles before breakfast get palpitations just thinking about doing curls or using a hyperextension machine.

I can't say I blame them. Gyms have long had a reputation for being strongholds of a certain kind of macho mentality. Then there's the notion, however false, that lifting weights makes you bigger and bulkier, which goes against everything women are taught to strive for in this carb-counting, calorie-obsessed, bleu-cheese-on-the-side culture of ours.

I truly believe that women more than understand the benefits of weight training in terms of appearance, long-term health, strength, and self-esteem, but often, finding enough free time is the greatest dilemma. Without question, lifting weights allows women to live longer, healthier, more robust lives, so if possible, please find the time, even if it's only 15 minutes to start with. I've seen how much it's helped my wife, Jennifer, who never worked out when we first met and now does it happily three times a week. Admittedly, she's one of those very lucky people who is very disciplined, and because of that she was able to drop nearly thirty pounds of pregnancy weight in mind-boggling time. But I'm amazed by how much more energy and physical strength she's developed since she started doing these exercises.

For many women in America, "working out" means going for a run or perhaps taking a health-club class like spinning, pilates, or kickboxing. Aerobics are great for burning calories, but women need *additional* forms of exercise to really stay strong. It's just a fact of physiology: women don't naturally develop as much muscle as men do because their set of hormones, and their smaller muscle fibers. To prove how much weight training can do, take two weeks and spend 45 minutes lifting weights instead of running on the treadmill. I promise, the benefits will be twentyfold.

At first, the tangible results of lifting are pretty obvious. It tones and builds a more fit and sensual overall appearance, improves mood, and lifts the energy level. And no, it doesn't make you look like Mrs. Olympia. Because women don't have the testosterone men have, it's impossible to develop the same sort of pronounced musculature. Instead, you improve posture, tighten soft spots, and accentuate curves in all the right places.

Strong muscles are also essential for keeping weight under control. The more muscle mass the body has, the faster it metabolizes food. In fact, building muscle can help a woman increase her metabolism by as much as 15 percent. The flip side is that without use, muscles shrink and the body burns fewer calories. Therefore, even if you eat exactly the same amount of food you did a few years earlier, you end up gaining weight. The sad truth is, an adult who doesn't do some sort of exercise loses 20 percent of muscle mass between the ages of 40 and 60. By age 90, a sedentary person has lost 70 percent of her overall ability to do everyday physical tasks.

But here's the amazing thing: A 65-year-old woman who exercises can be as fit as a 30-year-old woman who doesn't! And even a 90-year-old woman who's been exercising for years loses only about 30 percent of her functional ability.

When you lift weights, you don't just maintain muscle tissue; you actually increase the quality of the muscle fiber. The good news is, it's never too late to start lifting. Studies have found that even people who don't touch weights until their seventies or eighties show significant improvement in muscle strength, tone, and overall flexibility.

Weight training also reduces the risks of osteoporosis, since researchers believe that when a muscle contracts against resistance, the exertion actually increases bone density by stimulating cell growth. Likewise, strong muscles are better able to absorb the stress around joints, thereby fighting off arthritis.

I realize that lifting weights is an acquired taste, like liver pate—it takes a while to get used to it. So, if you don't have a fitness background, it's alienating, intimidating, completely daunting. Which is why it has to be approached casually. I don't care if you go to the gym for 15 minutes, touch a weight, and leave. You can even start by *watching* other people exercise on television. Whatever gets you into the mind-set. Just don't rush into it. That's probably the biggest mistake people make. They get sore and they never come back to the gym. Hang in there. I *promise* it's worth it.

What follows is a program that targets a woman's entire body, with particular emphasis on traditional trouble spots: the buttocks, hips, thighs, and belly. The way to use these exercises most effectively is to run through the entire workout three times a week, which should take about an hour each time once you get the hang of it. If you're not ready for the big commitment, start with one day a week and see how it feels. There's absolutely no need to rush. It took years to get out of shape. What's a few more weeks or months to get yourself back on track?

Finally, one of the biggest myths about fitness training is that you can work off weight or build strength in one particular area to the exclusion of other areas. I hear women talking about this all the time. "I just want to flatten my stomach." The truth is that spot reduction doesn't work. *Never has. Never will.* All these ads and exercise machines that promise flat stomachs and narrow waistlines are wasting your time. They're taking your money and laughing all the way to the bank. It's not right. Trust me when I say you can't just erase belly fat or slim your thighs except through liposuction. You need to work the *entire* body, not just one area, to get the results you want.

On the next few pages my wife, Jennifer, mother of three, will demonstrate what's worked for her.

★

★ CARDIO WARM-UP ★

The Move: You can of course use the cardio machine of your choice—but if women want to build up their buttocks, forget treadmills, it's a waste of effort. Use a rowing machine and get real cardio, fat-burning results and build the buttocks and shoulders at the same time. Five minutes is all you need, with minimum resistance.

Time: 5 minutes.

The Sly Report: The cardio warm-up is your opportunity to clear your head and leave the thoughts of the day behind. The next hour is your time to focus on yourself—and you deserve it. But remember: five minutes is all I'm asking. Your heart will be pounding plenty with the exercises to come.

TIP

Raise the incline or resistance levels to make your five minutes really count. Don't be afraid to work up a sweat.

THE TREADMILL: GOING NOWHERE FAST

People become treadmill maniacs and stairclimber junkies and think an aerobic workout is the only exercise they need to stay in shape. It's not. Sure, you're sweating and building endurance and losing weight, but you're not changing your strength. You're not building muscle. The only way you're really going to transform your body, the *only* way you can see serious improvements in your physique, is by lifting weights.

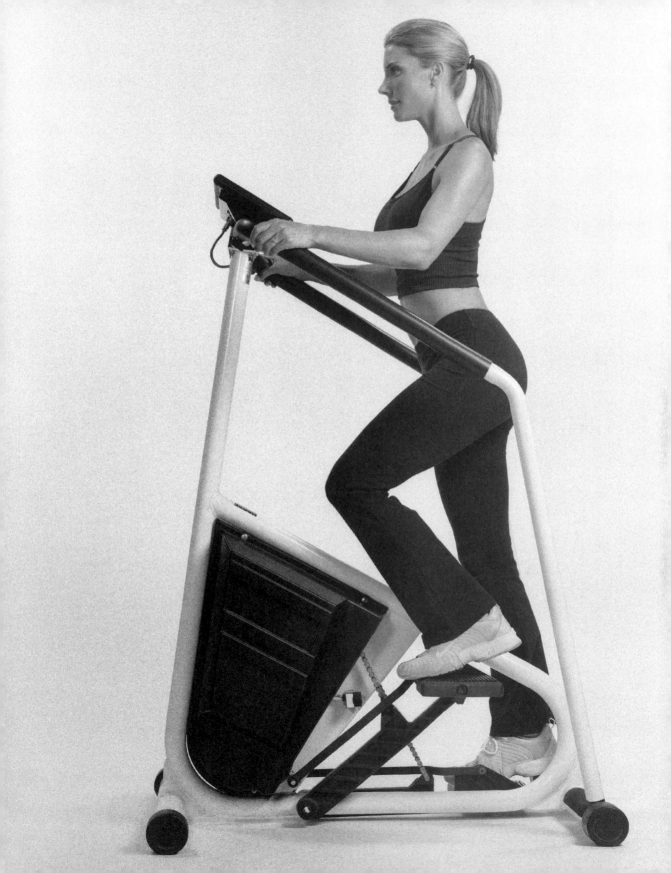

TIP

The mistake most people make is reaching forward toward the toes. Also, avoid any lunging motions, which could hurt your back. This should be a slow and smooth movement.

★ CRUNCHES ON A ★ FITNESS BALL
(abdominals)

The Move: With the ball centered at the small of your back and your feet comfortably apart for stability, reach straight up as if you are trying to grab a beam high above your chest. It's only an 8- to 10-inch movement and you should definitely feel it in your abs.

Sets: Work your way up to 3 sets of 10.

The Sly Report: Forget the upper abs. Your upper abs get exercise every time you pick something up or bend over. It's the lower abs that need special attention, and nothing does the trick quite like some time on the big rubber ball. The ball isn't just more comfortable than the floor, it also intensifies your workout. Balancing in that position brings the buttocks and thighs into play and requires the abs to be constantly engaged, so you never let up.

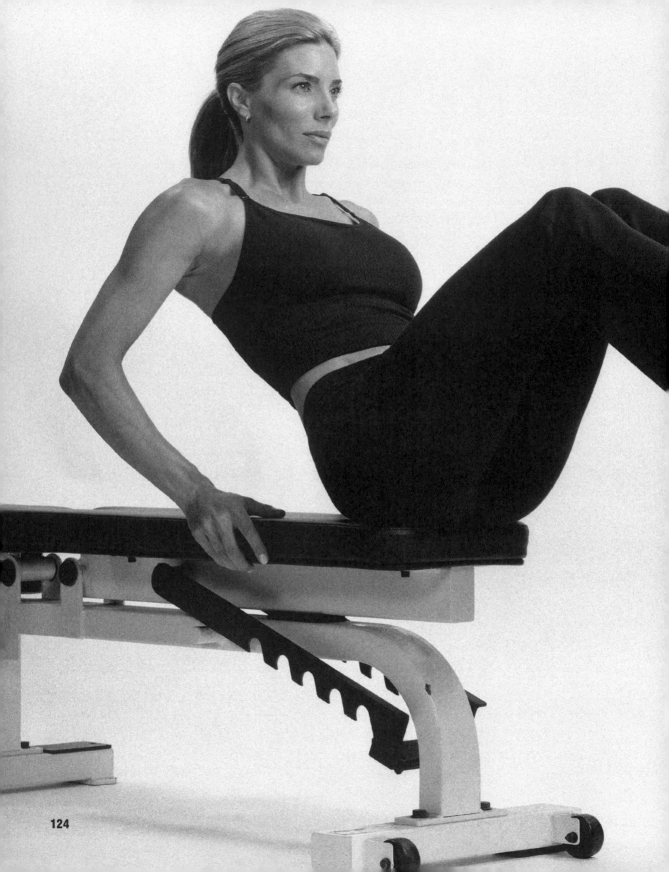

★ BENT KNEE RAISES ON A FLAT BENCH ★
(abdominals)

The Move: Sit at the far edge of a bench with your hands holding on behind you and your arms bent for support. Lean back slightly and slowly straighten your legs out in front of you. Bend your knees as you slowly bring them toward your chest as far as possible. Return to the starting position.

Sets: 2 sets of 10.

The Sly Report: This is a fantastic way to tighten up the lower abdominal muscles, which are the most ignored part of the abdominal wall. The lower abs are where gravity does the most damage, especially after a pregnancy or weight gain. Women are constantly looking for ways to get this area in shape. Look no further.

TIP
The key is to keep your back as straight as possible and at a 45-degree angle as you extend your legs. Just as important is to move slowly and breathe. You'll understand once you try it. Finally, avoid the common mistake of bringing the upper body to the knees rather than the knees to the upper body.

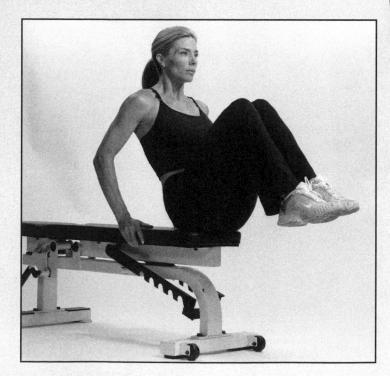

★ STOMACH VACUUM ★
(abdominals)

The Move: Stand with your hands on your hips and your feet comfortably apart. Inhale deeply from your diaphragm, pulling the stomach inward while squeezing your glutes. Hold your breath for five seconds and then slowly exhale for 10 seconds.

Sets: 2 sets of 6.

The Sly Report: Here's a great way to help your abdominal wall help itself. This move trains the stomach muscles to become shorter and therefore flatter. As you suck in your gut, imagine you're straightening up to kiss someone.

TIP
For variation, you can also try this move seated. Just keep your back straight.

★ INCLINE BENCH PRESS ★
(chest)

The Move: Lying back on the incline bench with a dumbbell in each hand, press both dumbbells straight up overhead from the base of the shoulders, your palms facing outward. Once the arms are fully extended, gently tap the dumbbells overhead before slowly returning the weights to the base of the shoulders. Inhale as you lower the weights, exhale as you press them up.

Sets: 2 sets of 10.

The Sly Report: Because women don't have the same amount of muscle on the breastbone as men, it's not worth overdoing it with chest exercises. This is the best one for women because it tightens the fleshy area between the shoulder and the chest, which tends to get soft.

TIP

Many people do this exercise halfway. They either forget to tap the weights at the top or don't lower the weights to the base of the shoulders. For the proper effect, get 'em all the way up and down on each rep.

★ INCLINE BENCH ★
DUMBBELL FLYS
(chest)

The Move: Lying back on an incline bench with dumbbells in each hand, bring the weights directly overhead, arms fully extended, palms facing each other. From this starting position, lower the dumbbells out to your sides, your arms opening wide as if you are about to give a hug. You'll feel the stretch across your rib cage into your arms. As you bring the weights back up, close the hug by following the natural arc back to the top, finishing overhead with the dumbbells touching.

Sets: 2 sets of 10.

The Sly Report: This exercise is another great upper chest workout, but it also works wonders for the shoulders, a sensuous but often neglected area. The shoulders create a beautiful silhouette and help your posture. When your shoulders are strong, you feel much more energetic and vital.

TIP

Slow and steady definitely win this race. Bring the weights down twice as slowly as you did pressing up. Be sure to maintain the arc motion over your chest rather than pressing, and don't exaggerate the stretch at the bottom of the exercise, or you could damage your shoulder joints. Never use heavy weights for this move.

★ PUNCHING ★ DUMBBELLS
(shoulders)

The Move: Holding a light dumbbell (two to five pounds) in each hand, stand in a comfortable position with one knee slightly forward and both knees slightly bent. Punch one arm straight out and bring it back, then punch the other arm out and bring it back. This should become a fluid motion and feel like you're taking normal punches.

Sets: Work up to 25 reps.

The Sly Report: A classic boxer's exercise, this one does unbelievable things for the trapezius, the shoulders, the biceps, and the grip. It also improves coordination, balance, and posture. It can be aerobic if you want it to be, and it's also fun (as exercises go).

TIP

Keep your arms up at shoulder height. For extra burn, punch in ultra-slow motion.

★ CABLE PRESS-DOWNS ★
(triceps)

The Move: Attach a short bent bar to a high cable machine. Facing the machine and keeping your back straight, take hold of the bar with an overhand grip and press it down from your midsection to your thighs. Then slowly release and let the bar come up as far as possible without moving your elbows until the weight returns to the starting position. Make sure your elbows are tight against your body and that your arms are fully extended at the bottom of the exercise.

Sets: 2 sets of 10.

The Sly Report: The triceps are a major trouble area for women. If you're not careful, the underside of your upper arms can get very loose as you get older. Biceps get a natural workout, since we lift things all day, but the *pushing* motion necessary to build great triceps usually only happens in the gym.

TIP
Avoid the temptation to bend forward. If you need some relief, bend slightly at the knees instead. You'll get the best results if you release the bar slowly from the bottom of the exercise.

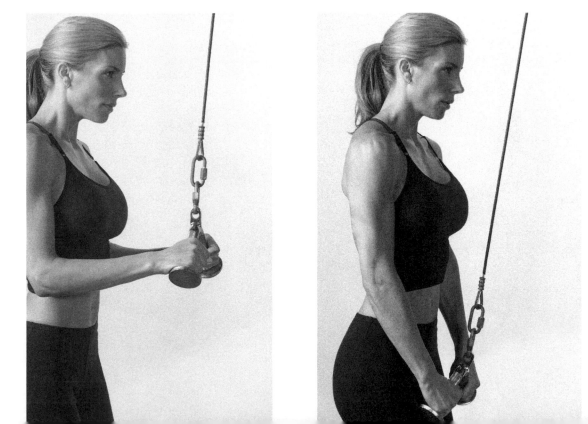

★ ONE-ARM ★ EXTENSIONS
(triceps)

The Move: In a comfortable standing position, hold a light dumbbell (two to five pounds) in one hand and raise it straight above you, keeping your upper arm close to your head. Slowly bring down the weight behind your head, lowering the dumbbell in a semicircular motion until your elbow points to the ceiling. Return to the starting position and repeat for your other arm. Your elbow and upper arm should move as little as possible.

Sets: 2 sets of 10.

The Sly Report: This is another stellar triceps exercise, and there's an almost meditative quality to it when it's done slowly, as it should be. The results are fantastic. Developed triceps are probably the surest sign that a woman is in great shape.

TIP
You can do this exercise standing or sitting. Just keep your back straight.

★ PUSH-UPS FROM THE KNEE ★
(triceps)

The Move: Lie flat on the floor with your hands palm-down next to each shoulder. Keeping your knees and feet on the ground, push up your body until your elbows lock. Slowly lower your upper body to the starting position. You should be looking straight out rather than down the entire time.

Sets: Work up to anywhere from 25 to 50 reps.

The Sly Report: Ah, good old push-ups. It's you and your body weight in an all-out effort to sculpt those oft-neglected triceps. I recommend doing these from the knees, at least in the beginning. It's really important to maintain a straight back and to keep the hands almost directly *under* the shoulders. Otherwise, this becomes a chest exercise. Remember to exhale as you push up and inhale on the way back down. Explode up, slow down.

TIP
Once you get comfortable with this, try regular push-ups.

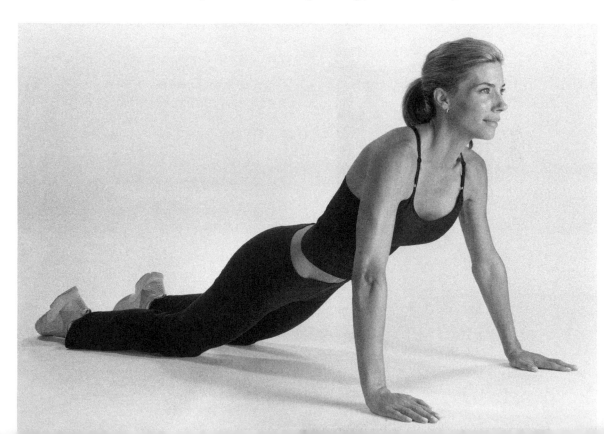

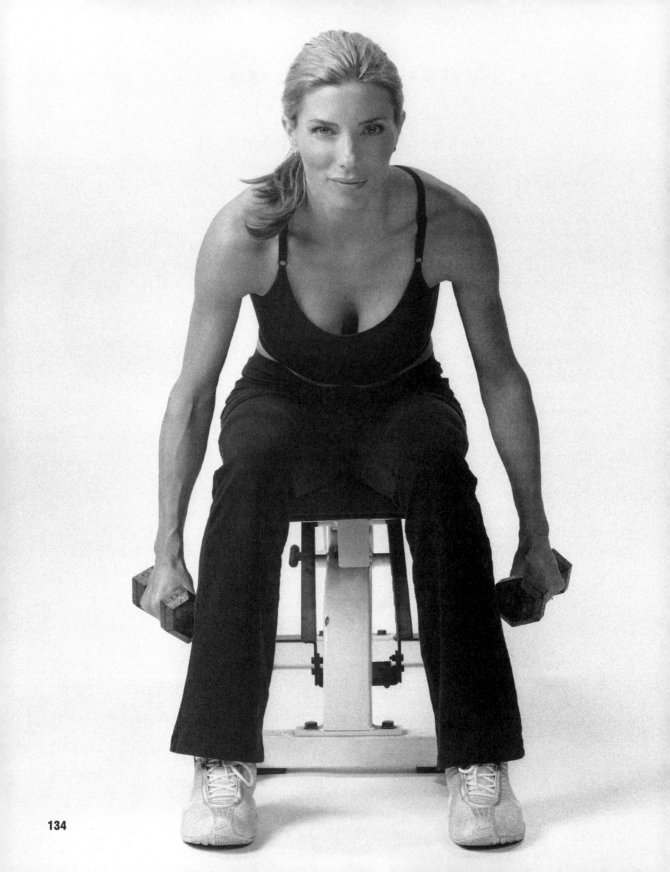

★ BENT-OVER LATERALS ★
(back—option A)

The Move: Sitting on the edge of a flat bench with a dumbbell in each hand and your hands at your sides, lean forward slightly and raise the dumbbells, pulling your arms apart until the dumbbells are in line with your shoulders. It should feel like you're lifting two jugs of water and pouring them out at the top. Slowly return the weights to your side in an arcing motion and repeat.

Sets: 2 sets of 10.

The Sly Report: Choose one of these three exercises for your back workout. They all do the trick. This one works the deltoids, the muscles that connect your back and shoulder muscles. Great for definition, women love this exercise because it makes you look great when you're showing off your shoulders and back in the summer. It certainly works with Jennifer. She puts me to shame.

TIP
Bend forward like you're cautiously peering over a steep cliff. In other words, a little but not too much.

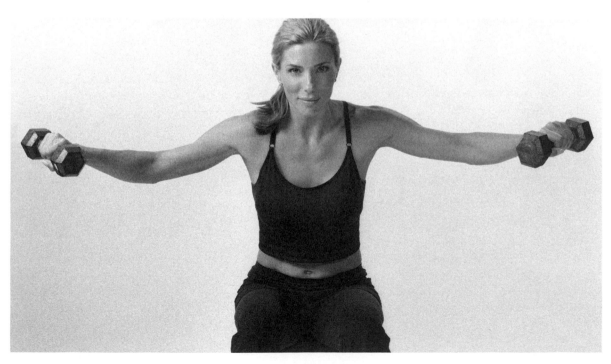

TIP

Again, you can alternate this option with the other two back exercises. As with all these moves, start with light weights to see how it feels. Keep the spine straight and don't lean forward or bend over at the end of each repetition.

★ SEATED ROWS ★
(back—option B)

The Move: As you're seated facing the machine, bend your knees and secure your feet on the foot plate. Grab hold of the pulley handle. Take a breath and pull the handle until it touches your lower rib cage. Slowly return the weights to the starting position, exhaling as you complete the move.

Sets: 2 sets of 10.

The Sly Report: I love this back exercise for women. It isolates all the major muscles of the back and helps strengthen your posture.

★ SEATED PULL-DOWNS ★
(back—option C)

The Move: As you're seated facing the machine, secure your thighs under the restraint pad. Grab hold of the overhead bar with a wide overhand grip. Take a breath and pull the bar down to the top of your chest. Slowly return the weights to the starting position, exhaling as you complete the move.

Sets: 2 sets of 10.

The Sly Report: This is the easiest of the three back moves and is probably the least helpful. However, it works the latissimus muscles of the central back and has some secondary benefits for the forearm and biceps, so it's worth adding to the mix occasionally.

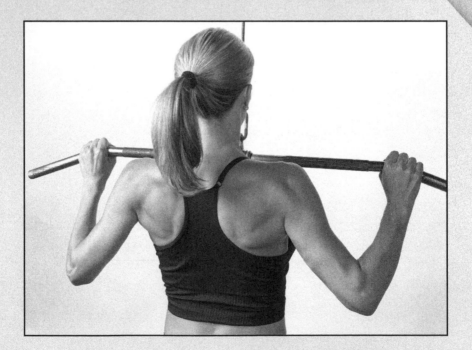

TIP

If you've ever wanted to do chin-ups but didn't have the strength, this machine will prepare you for the bar.

139

★ HALF-LUNGES ★
(buttocks and thighs)

The Move: Holding a flat bench for support, step forward with your left foot, keeping your back straight. Balance your weight evenly by bending your knees until the front leg is at a 90-degree angle and your back knee almost touches the floor. Hold that pose for a second and then return to the starting position by extending your front leg. Repeat this "lunge" movement with the opposite leg and then alternate legs. (See Sly's move for this on page 105.)

Sets: 2 sets of 10.

The Sly Report: This is one of those foolproof exercises that always gets results. My wife really relies on this one. You've heard of "cheeks of concrete"? This is the exercise.

TIP
Keep your back straight. Don't allow your knee to extend beyond your toes. If it does, take a wider stance. To make this work even better, hold two light dumbbells at your sides, palms facing in.

★ BENCH STEP UP ★
(buttocks and thighs)

The Move: Stand in front of a flat, secure bench and slowly step up, then back down. It should feel like you're climbing stairs three at a time.

Sets: 2 sets of 10.

The Sly Report: It looks easy, but this is definitely a power move. If you watch Olympic sprinters and hurdlers, you'll notice they have very developed butts. It's because they're constantly getting their knees up, and it's all about the push. I can't think of a better way to tone your glutes than by stepping up like this. Obviously, you don't even need a gym for this one. Take the stairs wherever you go.

TIP
The bench shouldn't be much higher than 18 inches. Straighten your back leg as you step up. For an extra lift, stand on your tiptoes for 2 seconds at the top.

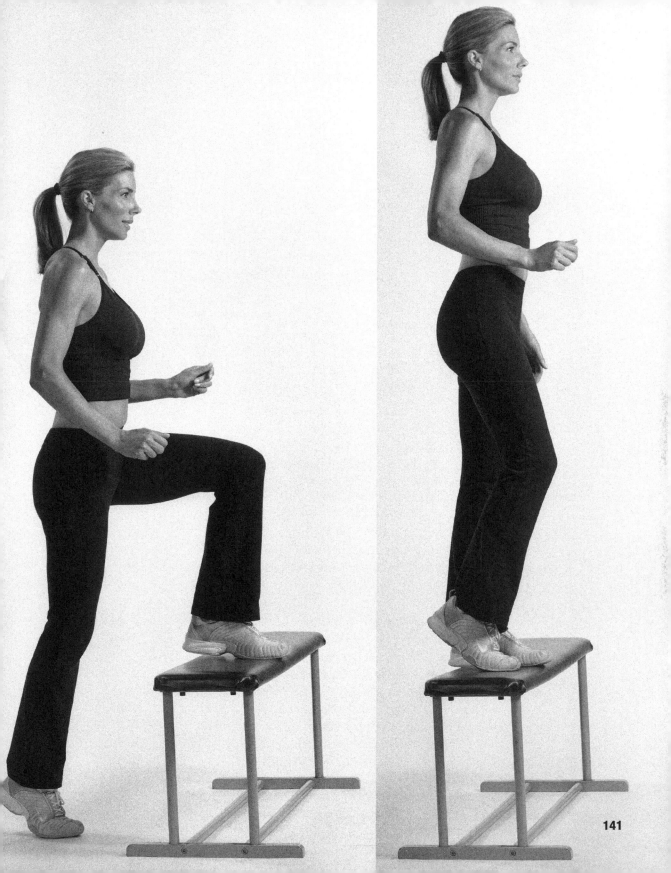

141

★ HYPEREXTENSIONS ★
(back and buttocks)

The Move: Lie facedown on a hyperextension or back-extension bench, securing your ankles under the ankle supports. Your upper thighs should lie flat across the main padding, leaving enough room for you to bend forward at the waist. Hold your hands behind your head or in front of you, or cross your arms at your chest. Slowly bend forward at the waist as far as you can while keeping your back flat. Then raise your upper body until your legs and torso are in a straight line again (arching up further can injure your back). Breathe out while you lower your torso and breathe in as you raise it.

Sets: 3 sets of 10.

The Sly Report: Hyperextensions are your butt's best friend. There is no better workout for the buttocks and lower back, and I must say it has a fantastic effect on women. The exercise causes the glutes to go into extreme contraction, which has a pumping effect on the upper part of the buttocks. If you stay the course, the results will be truly remarkable and in a short period of time.

TIP
Once you get the hang of this, try holding a barbell plate in your arms to increase the overall effect.

★ CARDIO FINALE ★

The Move: Split this exercise between two cardio machines of your choice to get your heart rate up to between 125 and 150 beats per minute. Build to an intensity level of 8 or 9 out of 10.

Time: 10 minutes on each machine.

The Sly Report: Ending your workout with a big cardio push helps flush out the toxins and relieve any tension built up over the last 40 minutes. Let 'em see you sweat!

TIP

Once you've graduated from the rowing machine, try the VersaClimber, which simulates the effect of scurrying up a ladder. Used with gusto, it's the mack daddy of cardio machines.

Final Word: Do the same workout for at least one month straight, three days a week, Monday, Wednesday, and Friday. I suggest you have a protein drink or a "good" carb snack before a workout. But never go into a workout with an empty tank.

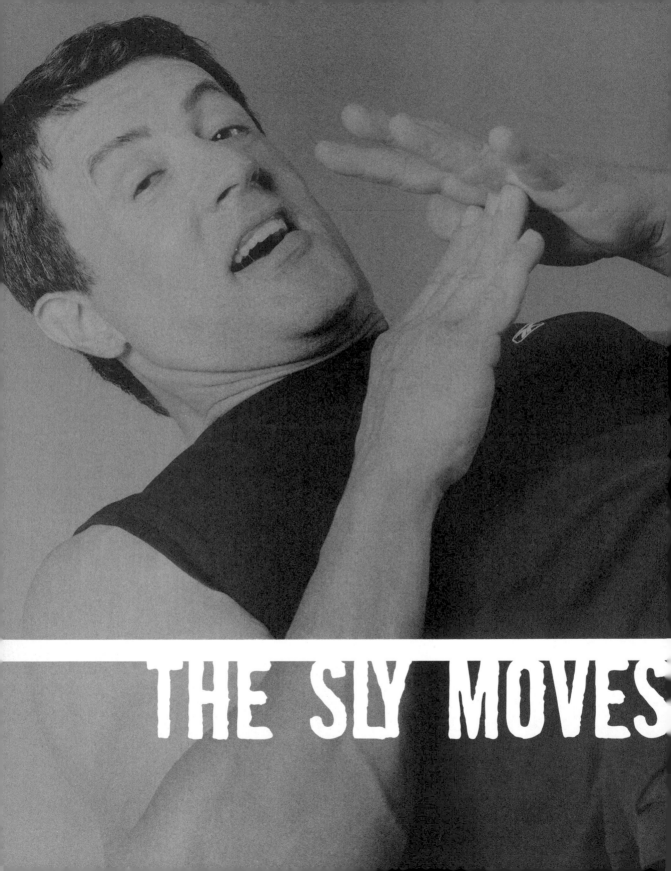

THE SLY MOVES

PART 3

EATING PLAN

Let's get one thing out of the way up front: *Diets don't work forever!* Believe me, I've tried them all. Atkins, Pritikin, the Zone, watermelon, seeds, macro, cottage cheese, grapefruit, cabbage soup. At various points, I've eaten only chicken, only meat, only vegetables, and only yogurt. And I've frequently relied on a Greek fisherman's diet: all seafood all the time. I've tried low carbs, no carbs, high-altitude low carbs (for *Cliffhanger*), even mountain climber high-altitude high carbs (the Swiss chocolate and cheese diet).

A new diet is like a new romance. Every time you start one, the results are different, exciting, sometimes intense, and the diets promise that they'll always be there for you, always care for you. And you believe it with your whole being. Then the passion begins to cool along with the promise that Mr. Diet will take all your worries away. You got taken because you wanted so badly to believe.

Look, any diet will work *for a while*. I could put you on a limited whipped cream diet and you'd lose weight if you were served during certain times of the day and stayed physically active. It's like that guy who ate all those Subway sandwiches and dropped 245 pounds. He put his mind to it, exercised every day, reduced his overall calorie intake, and followed a regimented plan. The pounds are going to come off that way. If you stop eating just one slice of bread a day, *one*, you'll lose 8 to 10 pounds a year doing nothing else.

It bothers me to see so many people out there cutting carbohydrates out of their diet. The high-protein, low-carb craze is nothing but a setup for frustration and failure, not to mention all sorts of potential health problems. Our bodies need carbohydrates, we crave them, and if we slash them out of our lives, we're just asking for trouble. Plus, answer this: If the Atkins, South Beach, and other diets work so well, why can't most of us name five people on them who've lost weight *and kept the weight off* for a year or more? It just doesn't happen! For every 100 people who lose weight, a whopping 95 will gain it back *and add more*.

SAY GOOD-BYE TO DIETING

About 20 years ago, I stopped dieting completely and I've never been healthier. Don't get me wrong. I still watch what I eat. I'm not snacking on cupcakes and ice cream all day (though I still indulge in those pleasures regularly). It's just that I don't think of what I do as "dieting." I eat what I eat and know how to regulate it.

If I gain five pounds, I'll just subtract some of my regular foods—usually in the carbohydrate department—until the weight comes off. If I'm aiming to get stronger or add muscle, I know exactly which combination of proteins, carbs, and fats will take me there. There's no big secret. For me, quality nutrition comes down to common sense, a little bit of willpower, and simplicity.

Deep down inside, everybody knows how to eat smart. Our brains have a wonderful little sensor called the appestat, which distinguishes good food from bad. I can take 1,000 people into a supermarket and tell them to pick out healthy foods and unhealthy foods and every one will know the difference. Green and leafy, nutritious. Glazed and powdery, not. We know that and yet our behavior doesn't reflect that. Why? Are we looking for food to free us from stress? To make us feel less lonely? To make us happy?

People give food such power over their lives. I know because I've done it myself. It's one of the hardest things to change. If you obsess over food the way you obsess over a loved one, it's time to retool that dynamic. I've gotten to a point where food is almost secondary in my life. It really is. And maybe I'm an exception, but I can't tell you how strong it makes me, knowing I've freed myself from that habit.

How did I do it? Common sense, a little bit of willpower, and simplicity.

Let's talk about simplicity for a minute. I've eaten the same basic foods all my life. Everyone's a creature of habit when it comes to food. People enjoy the foods they enjoy and it's hard to break that pattern. Think about it. When you go to a restaurant, don't you usually order one of the same three or four basic dishes every time or a slight variation on them? I feel the same way about eating smart. *You find a few foods you like, that you've been raised with, that you feel comfortable with, hopefully that are good for you, and those become your go-to foods.*

Unfortunately, it's easy to go to some very unhealthy places these days, which is why some of us need to make changes in what we eat. Just walk through any supermarket in America. Shelves are crammed with cheap, mass-produced, and highly processed foods that explode with calories by design, what I believe is an absolute conspiratorial plan by many food companies to hook children on their incredibly unhealthy products. Thousands upon thousands of kids become addicted to sugary soft drinks and toxic snack foods before they even get to nursery school. As part of a national pastime, we drive-thru and supersize and all-we-can-eat and still "find room" for the double-fudge chocolate blackout cake. *Chemicals are added that actually increase our appetites.*

Two-thirds of U.S. adults are officially overweight and roughly half of those have upgraded to full-on obesity. In the past decade alone, there's been a 7 to 10-pound average weight gain across the American population. Worldwide, the number of obese people swelled from 200 million in 1995 to 300 million in 2003 and 1.7 billion of the planet's 6 billion inhabitants are considered overweight. In 2003 alone, U.S. taxpayers footed the bill for more than $75 billion in obesity-related medical costs. This year in America, there will be 400,000 deaths associated with being overweight. *To not gain weight in America today is almost an impossibility.*

If you see yourself among those statistics, do not panic. In fact, be kind to yourself. The more you try to "diet" and starve yourself, the more you're going to lose control and snap back in the other direction and binge. So many people have all this guilt because they couldn't stick to a diet. They blame themselves for not going the distance. In fact, it's almost always the diet that's the problem. It's the diet that's too restrictive or too boring or contrary to the principles of good nutrition. It's not your fault at all.

And here's the good news. Even slight variations in how you eat can make huge improvements in how you look and feel. Substituting whole grain for white bread, honey for sugar, olive oil for fattening dressings, or even just taking *half* as many bites of that daily cookie or cheeseburger will make an enormous difference in your overall well-being. Just do the math. If you eliminate just 100 calories a day by skipping a handful of pretzels or a light beer, that's 700 calories a week, which cuts out about *10 pounds a year*. If you don't think that's a lot, hold a 10-pound weight over your head for a minute or two.

Diets do nothing but rob us of our dignity. They tell us we're too fat, we're eating the wrong foods, we're unhealthy, we're going to die. Who needs that? I think we need to accept who we are, learn to love our cravings, and find inspiration in small improvements rather than in unrealistic goals.

SAY IT ONCE AND SAY IT LOUD, "I'M BIG BUT STRONG"

In my opinion, big is here to stay. It's naive to think we're going to "cure" obesity or tighten the collective waistline of nearly 2 billion overweight people. At this point, it's next to impossible. With remote controls and elevators and the Internet and video games, we've practically engineered physical activity out of our daily lives. Our meal portions have grown to Flintstones-like proportions. Airplane seats no longer accommodate the standard derriere. But unless we discover some kind of cheap weight pill, an outbreak of skinny just isn't going to happen.

I'm here to tell you it's okay to be big if you just try to *stay strong*. Even when I was watching my weight for various roles, I always gave myself permission occasionally to break out the breads, pastas, and even the donuts and ice cream. I just did it intelligently. We'll get to my actual meal plans later in this section, but first I want to explore this idea of being big *and* strong.

I've always thought you need a little meat on your bones to be healthy and to look good, especially as you get older. People are always talking about getting "back to their high school weight" or fitting into their wedding dresses. The fact is, those are misguided goals. We actually need some extra weight as we age. Look at people in their seventies, eighties and nineties who are rail-thin as opposed to those who are a bit more full-faced. They're gaunt. Sickly-looking. Who looks healthier? My advice to a lot of people is: Gain ten pounds, you'll look better.

There's plenty of science to back me up on this one. Some of the country's leading physiologists and nutritionists are discovering that exercising and eating smarter are more important to long-term health than losing weight. After studying more than 35,000 adults, the Cooper Institute, a Dallas-based center that researches fitness habits and health, concluded that a physically active life prevents the illnesses typically attributed to overweight people—such as type-II diabetes, heart disease, and cancer—even in people considered extremely obese. *At the same time, the death rate among men of average weight who were not fit was more than double that of obese men who were fit.* That bears repeating. The overweight guys who exercised regularly outlived the skinny ones who didn't—by a ratio of 2 to 1.

After tracking nearly 1,000 mostly overweight women for four years, a 2004 study from the University of Florida found that the overweight women who were at least moderately active were far less likely to develop heart disease and related problems than the women who were inactive.

What this tells us is we all have a fighting chance. You might be 450 pounds, but if you get off the couch right now and walk a few hundred steps to the corner and back, you're that much closer to feeling good about yourself. If you're addicted to chocolate cookie dough ice cream, have it! Just eliminate something else from your diet the next day. You've improved your life almost without even trying. I've already shared my exercise secrets with you, but for now, even just a few extra stairs or a few more minutes sweeping the porch will start to make a difference. Staying in motion is the key.

I know being overweight is not easy for some people. We live in a society where thin is in and where physical appearance matters as much if not more than good health. Everyone everywhere is searching for that one regimen, that one book, that one magic pill that will shed pounds and keep them off. If CNN told us tomorrow that eating wood would take three inches off the waist, a million people would go out tomorrow and start gnawing on oak trees. Until the next fad came along.

It's so easy to get caught up in that cycle and it's even easier to let it depress you. I can put on weight as fast as anybody, believe me. I recently went to Germany and in seven days gained seven pounds. Then I came home and got back on the program. Not to get skinny, not to reach some cultural "ideal." That's not going to happen. But to get to a weight *I* can live with.

WHERE TO BEGIN

I don't consider myself a genetic freak. My metabolism isn't high, it isn't low; it's right in the middle. I gain weight and lose weight just like everyone else, and battling the bulge is a fight I wage every day. But I accept that, and as we get into this program, that's all I ask of you. Accept who you are, accept your weaknesses and your frustrations, accept that you'll have cravings and setbacks and that you will fail. But above all, accept that every day's a new opportunity to try again. Sure, you're going to slip up. Just start again the next day until it begins to sink in and becomes a habit.

SLY WEIGHS IN ON THE DIETS

Is anyone out there *not* obsessed with a diet these days? Weight loss and nutrition books more than doubled their share of overall book sales between 2002 and 2003. With so many programs and promises (not to mention those incredible 12-week "before-and-after" pictures. Yeah, right!), it's easy to be seduced. But while some diets work better than others, almost all the popular ones focus on short-term gains rather than true lifelong success. Here's my take on a few key diets, but consider the source. Is the preacher practicing what he is preaching? Look at the cover. *Does he or she have the body to back up his or her message? If not, why on earth would anybody trust what that person says?*

DR. ATKINS' NEW DIET REVOLUTION by Robert Atkins, M.D.

Steaks with blue cheese. Bacon double cheeseburgers without the bun. Bacon and eggs and bacon and eggs and bacon and . . .

The now-classic Atkins diet urges you to cut carbohydrates while upping the amount of proteins without worrying about fats. The theory goes that since our bodies burn carbs before fat, it's more efficient to simply lose the carbs in the first place.

I like to think of Atkins as the caveman diet, because you end up eating meats, meats, and more meats. No question, the high-protein, low-carb approach sheds pounds, especially if you combine it with a regular fitness plan, but it's far from flawless and may even lead to serious health problems. There's a reason people are now abandoning this diet in droves.

I've tried it. My problem was that I started to practically feel the grease pulsating through my arteries after a few weeks. All that saturated fat has to go somewhere, and your veins and arteries are the first place it visits, putting millions of people at risk for heart disease. Plus, I have issues with processed meats, which this diet allows, with all the additives and preservatives.

Atkins is also the least sexy diet I can think of. People who are on it too long develop what I call "Atkins face," that gaunt, sickly look you get when the protein burns the subcutaneous fat around the cheeks and mouth. Because it's low on fiber, it makes you constipated. Many people say it causes headaches, and because of the release of ketones, a waste product of fat, it leads to bad breath.

BODY FOR LIFE by Bill Phillips

I know Bill Phillips. We've worked together in the past. I agree with a lot of what he says. His book is packed with good old-fashioned fundamentals. But some of it is *way* too good to be true.

Phillips's basic idea is that six small meals a day keeps the fat away. When you eat the standard three square meals, your body tends to store unburned calories as body fat. But when you graze all day long, as part of an active lifestyle, you accelerate metabolism and maintain consistent energy levels. I'm all for that as long as the process doesn't take over your life.

My main complaint is Bill's implication that you can get mega-results in just 12 weeks. It is completely impossible unless—and this is important—you had an excellent body before you gained the weight. Muscle memory is a powerful thing, and people who've been ripped can do it again in less time. But for most of us, that's a nonissue. Maybe it's just me, but in the first *Rocky*, I took supplements and worked out for six months, five hours a day, six days a week, and I never got a body like the one featured at the front of Bill's book—and I was under the watchful eye of boxing trainers and anxious studio executives. It took me from *Rocky* in 1975 until *Rocky III* in 1981 to get my "after" body.

THE SOUTH BEACH DIET by Arthur Agatston, M.D.

Agatston is a cardiologist who worked with some fancy Miami restaurateurs to come up with meal plans that are pretty solid. That is, if you happen to be a professional chef. Who in their right mind is going to julienne small red peppers for the Cod en Papillote? I mean, does anyone actually have time to peel and sauté the pound of yucca for the Roast Chicken with Sweet Garlic, Melted Onions and Sour Orange recipe? And let's not even talk about the Asian Grilled Tempeh Triangles or the Spanish Spiced

Rubbed Chicken with Mustard-Green Onion Sauce or the Grilled Filet Mignon with Roasted Garlic and Chipotle Pepper Chimichurri. This isn't a diet. It's a life sentence in the kitchen.

Finally, if you look at some editions of the book, it proclaims the ultimate lie on the cover: "Lose belly fat first!" Nonsense! *Again, there's no such thing as "spot" weight loss, just as there's no such thing as spot training in the gym.* When you lose weight, you *must* lose it all over your body, not just in one place.

PROTEIN POWER by Michael R. Eades, M.D.

You don't need a medical degree to get through the best-selling *Protein Power*, but it certainly helps. Eades gets deep inside the science of proteins, with pages and pages devoted to subjects like arachidonic acid and eicosanoids and hyperinsulinemia. His basic message is that a protein-rich, moderate-fat, low-carbohydrate diet will have you feeling better within a week.

The jury is still out on whether lots of protein is safe over the long term, but I'm dubious of any program that's deficient in essential nutrients from carbohydrates, fibers, and fruits. When a diet cuts out so many foods, it's almost impossible to sustain over the long term. And even with a moderately high-protein diet like this, you'll notice you don't eliminate the toxins from the body the way you should.

Finally, you may look stronger on a protein diet, but you're actually weaker. The muscles may get bigger, but there's no carbohydrate stream to deliver energy to them. You'll never have the same kind of endurance or bounce in your step that you get from a more balanced diet. I see this with boxers all the time. When I go to fights, I'll see one boxer who is totally shredded, with no more than 4 percent body fat and chiseled down to the bone. I can tell he's all about protein. But if his opponent is a little smoother, a little less defined, that's the guy I'm betting on. Most likely, the less chiseled fighter has been training with a mix of proteins and carbohydrates and will last longer. Mr. Protein may prevail in the earlier rounds, but count on the other guy to go the distance.

WEIGHT WATCHERS

Weight Watchers in theory is a fantastic idea and it's worked just fine for people who have been addicted to eating. There's something comforting about the group gatherings—like a warm inviting fire in a very dark, cold world. The trouble is, a lot of people find it difficult to build their life around tallying points and slipping away to meetings. I think if you have a simple plan and a place to go that encourages you regularly to stay in shape, such as a gym you like, you've got all you need.

THE PRITIKIN WEIGHT LOSS BREAKTHROUGH by Robert Pritikin

The Pritikin diet has been around for more than 20 years, and most people have heard of it even if they haven't tried it. My wife and I went on this diet about 10 years ago. We were in Aspen skiing and eating a lot of very good carbohydrates, a lot of fruit and vegetables, and I lost about 10 pounds immediately. I was impressed. Then I lost all my muscle tone. I became like a rubber band man, my arms felt weak and my body untoned. Next.

I honestly believe that when animal proteins are reduced, you become flabby and soft. Your body starts begging, "Feed me." It's as though you're depriving the body of something essential for philosophical or supposed health reasons. "Chicken is full of drugs and it's filthy," they'll tell you. But it's not the chicken, it's how the chicken is raised or prepared. You could eat a raw chicken right now and not get sick if it came from a farm where quality matters.

THE ZONE by Barry Sears, Ph.D.

Sears, a former MIT biochemical researcher, argues that the correct ratio of protein to fat to carbs should remain at a steady 30:30:40. That way, you're sure to maintain healthy insulin levels.

There's nothing revolutionary here. We've known forever that a balanced diet is key to good health. Some people complain that the Zone is too low in whole grains and calcium. And almost everyone agrees the program is way too complicated, with its "blocks" of food you need to multiply by three-quarters.

But the strangest part of the Zone is what Sears calls the "eyeball method." Portion sizes are based on the size of your hand. So in theory, if you have small hands, you could starve. If you're Shaquille O'Neal, you're golden. Seriously, the whole thing gets complicated pretty quickly. Protein should be the size of the palm of your hand, but carbohydrates should be the size of your fist. That is, unless they're "good" carbohydrates; then you're allowed two fistfuls. The five fingers of your hand should remind you to eat at least five times a day: three meals and two snacks.

Remember, any diet will get you results—for a while. You'll lose pounds at first, but unless your diet is simple and sensible and tailored specifically for your individual needs, it will eventually fail over the long haul.

THE MEDITERRANEAN DIET by Marissa Cloutier, M.S., R.D., and Eve Adamson

Traditional Mediterranean cuisine is one of the tastiest and most satisfying diets in the world as well as one of the healthiest. It helps lower rates of coronary heart disease and other chronic conditions, including diabetes and cancer.

A famous 1950 Stanford University study originally conducted to see if the Greeks could improve their diet after World War II concluded that the diet couldn't get much better. For more than 40 centuries, the Mediterraneans have thrived on a diet rich in whole grains, legumes, fruits, nuts, and seasonal vegetables, along with moderate amounts of dairy, fish, lamb, and occasional red meat. Since olive oil is the primary source of fat, the diet is low in cholesterol and saturated fats, which explains the low incidence of heart disease. And who can argue with a diet that encourages you to drink a little red wine?

As diets go, I like the Mediterranean diet. But again, it's a program that eventually will fail, unless people are willing to completely abandon American tastes for European ones.

EATING SMART WITH SLY MOVES

I've basically eaten the same foods for most of my life. Sure, I try something different occasionally or add new items depending on what's in season. I also give myself total freedom one day a week to eat whatever I want—ice cream, cheesecake, and especially the giant waffles Jennifer whips up on Sunday mornings. But to stay healthy and keep my body in shape, I always come back to the basics. *Always.*

Nutritionists tell us that simplicity and consistency are essential in controlling body weight over the course of a lifetime. It's certainly worked for me and it will work for you, too, particularly if you've failed on diets in the past. So many people have shame, guilt, and frustration about dieting. They blame themselves for not being strong enough to go the distance. But here's the thing. Almost always, *it's the diet's fault*. Over the long haul, most diets are just too difficult or restrictive to follow.

What follows is not a diet. It's simply a look at what people who truly enjoy eating can accomplish when they have a goal! John Travolta lost over 40 pounds to play a professional dancer when I directed him in the film *Staying Alive*. We discussed diet changes and an exercise regimen handled by a wonderful trainer named Dan Issacson, and in a short time, John had developed one of the *best Hollywood bodies in history.*

EATING SEVERAL TIMES A DAY

I think the smartest way to eat is to have three meals and two snacks throughout the day. And while most of the fad diets out there try to sustain you on 800 to 1,200 calories a day, I think that is nearly impossible by today's standards. You can lose weight on 1,800 to 2,000 a day and even a little more if you're knocking yourself out in the gym. Staying in shape is challenging enough. We don't need to starve ourselves, too. I recommend three regular meals to give you the fuel you need and three satisfying snacks to keep the edge off and the blood sugar and glycogen levels up.

The trend is to load up on protein and lay off the carbs. But unless you're an Olympic-bound athlete or a professional bodybuilder, there's absolutely *no* reason for it. If 80 percent of your diet is protein, which is

THE FOOD BASICS

These are the basics, the foods I've counted on for decades to manage my weight and keep me in shape. It's the simplest and only proven way I know to maintain a consistent, enjoyable, and nourishing approach to eating. Here's how to do it: have one protein, one or two carbs, and, for lunch and dinner, one vegetable. I also add small amounts of healthy fats to each meal, like good oils, seeds, and nuts. You'll find menus for some of my favorite meals at the end of this section. In the meantime, enjoy!

PROTEINS

Egg whites	Chicken	Scallops
Lean ham	Turkey breast	Shrimp
New York strip steak	Veal	Eggs
Lean pork	Flounder	Cottage cheese
Lean ground beef	Tuna	Italian sausage
Lean ground turkey	Crab	Mussels
	Lobster	Salmon

CARBOHYDRATES

Sweet potato	Yams	Peaches
Baked potato	Beets	Bananas
Whole grain pasta	Whole grain bread	Blueberries
Natural oatmeal	Apples	Figs
Shredded wheat	Melon	Dates
Steamed brown rice	Strawberries	Prunes
	Grapes	Pineapple

VEGETABLES

Asparagus	Cucumber	Cauliflower
Bell pepper	Beets	Green pepper
Broccoli	Mushroom	Avocado
Spinach	Eggplant	Peas
Corn	Beans	String beans
Tomato	Brussels sprouts	
	Dark green lettuce	

what many of the popular diet books recommend, you're setting yourself up for a heart attack.

I keep the ratio around 50–60 percent carbohydrate, 30 percent protein, and 20 percent good fats. It's pretty easy to remember, actually. When you look down at your plate, a little more than half should be vegetables and some good starches like brown rice or whole-wheat pasta, a third should be your main protein source, and the rest healthy fats such as olive oil. That may sound like a lot of carbohydrates, but carbs are much more enjoyable than high protein, and provide much more energy when you're exercising. And you will be exercising, right?

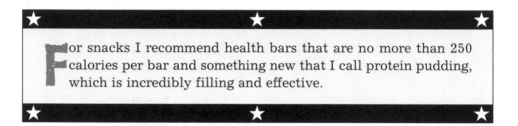

For snacks I recommend health bars that are no more than 250 calories per bar and something new that I call protein pudding, which is incredibly filling and effective.

THE CARBOHYDRATE FAIRY TALE

Once upon a time, a clever prince popularized the idea that eating fewer carbohydrates and more protein was the secret to having a great body. This determined young man—let's call him, oh, Dr. Fatkins—saw his kingdom grow (not to mention his coffers) as his enthralled subjects said goodbye to breads, rice, and pastas and hello to bacon double cheeseburgers without the bun.

That's about where our fairy tale ends. There's no "happily ever after" on a low-carb, high-protein diet. All you get are short-term fixes and long-range problems. In the first few weeks, people lose tons of weight, which is why it's so popular. But down the road, it actually makes you fatter and may even cause the sort of health problems all the king's men couldn't fix.

First, consider how low-carb, high-protein diets work. By cutting out virtually all carbohydrates from your diet and increasing your protein and fat, you trick the body into thinking it's starving. Without those energy-

BREAKING THE BREAD HABIT

My daughters wouldn't even consider having eggs without a couple pieces of toast. But if you're watching your weight, you'll need to cut back on how much bread you consume, especially if you're eating a lot of white bread or anything made with "refined" or "enriched" flour. Save the bread overload for the weekend, when you allow yourself to let it all go.°

The refining process removes the bran fiber and nutrient-rich germ from the grain, which makes bread lighter, whiter, and sweeter. But it also strips grains of essential vitamins E and B, iron, selenium, and other disease-fighting components. And without fiber, these grains turn to glucose and enter the bloodstream much faster than unrefined grains. Enriched grains are simply refined grains with certain nutrients—like niacin, riboflavin, thiamin, and iron—added back in. The trouble is, enrichment doesn't restore insoluble fiber and other beneficial ingredients that are lost during the milling process.

Whole grains are always the healthier option. With their fiber intact, carbohydrates are not absorbed as quickly into the bloodstream, which helps regulate blood sugar and keeps you feeling satiated longer. The unprocessed grains are rich in vitamins and minerals and full of fiber, which improves digestion.

Just be careful. Marketers have figured out all sorts of ways to disguise cheaper, sweeter refined grains. Just because bread is brown and has seeds or flecks of wheat doesn't mean it's whole grain. Nor is it whole grain if it's labeled multigrain, cracked wheat, seven-grain, twelve-grain, stone-ground, or 100 percent wheat.

providing carbs around, the body begins burning stores of glucose in the muscles and liver to get the fuel it needs. At the same time, because every gram of carbohydrate consumed causes the body to hold 2.4 grams of water, every carb you skip makes the body a few drops lighter. *The result: you lose muscle, you lose water, you lose weight.*

That's where the trouble begins. Losing precious lean muscle mass causes you to gain more weight. Here's why: Metabolically speaking, muscle tissue is active, which means it burns calories even when you're sitting around. Take away that active muscle and the body thinks it needs fewer calories to maintain your base weight. The body develops a new concept of how much it needs, and your old "normal" is now overeating. *That's why so many people put on pounds once they go off the diet.* On top of that, since it's so hard to rebuild muscle tissue, the weight you gain back is primarily fat. So not only are you heavier, you're actually weaker and less firm.

But wait, there's more. By doing away with carbohydrates like fruits, vegetables and grains, the body can't *function* properly. Your digestive system doesn't operate as efficiently and you lose essential nutrients and vitamins. Likewise, by increasing the fat, particularly saturated fat, with all that meat consumption, you're increasing your chances of developing cardiovascular problems.

Then there's "ketosis." When the body relies on stored muscle tissue for energy, it produces compounds called ketone bodies, a carbon waste product of fat. If you've tried the Atkins or South Beach diets, you probably knew you'd entered ketosis when you developed a slight buzz or got bomb breath. The problem is, the body can't live with ketones, which means the liver and kidney must work overtime to eliminate them. You may experience side effects—nausea, constipation, fatigue, headaches, dizziness, insomnia, depression, and irritability. Because ketosis makes the blood more acidic, it can, in the long term, reduce calcium absorption, which may lower bone density and cause kidney stones.

GOOD CARB, BAD CARB

Carbohydrates get absolutely no respect anymore. It's almost like there's a worldwide conspiracy against them. Television and magazines are loaded with anticarb advertisements, and even fast-food chains are betraying their allegiance to the noble energy source. Come on! What's the point of a bunless burger?

The truth is, all carbohydrates are not created equal. Yes, there are bad carbs. But there are also very good carbs, which serve as the body's favored fuel source.

We hardly need to be reminded of the bad carbs. Those are the processed ones that are low on fiber and deliver a quick jolt to your blood sugar levels. Once the blood sugar level drops, usually an hour or so later, the body starts craving more and more carbohydrates. It's that yo-yo cycle that causes people to eat and overeat.

Bad carbs are easy to identify. They taste addictive and they're often dressed in white. White flour and sugar are two of the biggest culprits, which means that white bread, syrups, toppings, frostings, most dressings, sugary soft drinks, cereals, and candy are best (though very difficult) to avoid. The same goes for anything fried. Skip white rice, too. It's so low in fiber, it's not worth stuffing a mattress with (there's a reason they throw it at weddings). And remember, sugar often hides on ingredient lists under the suffix "ose," like fructose or cellulose. Not that you need a label to tell you when you've eaten bad carbs. Your body will tell you. You'll either be hungry or asleep an hour or so later.

I practically lived on bad carbs in my early days, training for *The Lords of Flatbush* and even the first *Rocky*. But once I realized the other side of the carbohydrate story, my whole way of eating turned around.

Good carbohydrates, including nutrient-rich fruits and vegetables, are the body's absolute best sources for vitamins, fiber, and the antioxidants that help fight disease. What many people don't realize is that these good carbohydrates actually help you lose weight, since they help slow down the absorption of food and don't have the same roller-coaster effect on blood sugar levels that bad carbs do. The result is that good carbs keep you feeling full much longer after a meal.

You'll find good carbohydrates in whole grain breads and whole wheat pastas and brown rice, as well as fruits and vegetables. Start out your day with unprocessed oatmeal and see how much better you feel than when you have a regular bowl of sugar cereal. It's astonishing.

Some of my favorite good carbs are sweet potatoes, beets, and eggplant, which to me is the filet mignon of the vegetable world. You know you've eaten good carbs when you have a high energy level all day long.

The tasty "bad" carbs can be consumed on your free day and a half, so cheer up.

PROTEIN: PROS AND CONS

Most Westerners have way too much protein in their diets. North Americans and Western Europeans typically consume as much as double the amount of protein recommended by the World Health Organization. If more than 30 percent of your daily caloric intake is protein, you're over the limit.

What's considered protein? Here's an easy reminder: Anything that comes from the earth is a carb. Anything with a face is protein. Turkey, salmon, pheasant, escargot—they're all proteins.

Protein is vital for building muscles, bones, skin, hair, and blood. It helps the body fight infection, build and repair tissues, synthesize hormones and enzymes, and maintain a balance of fluids. You need protein to keep your muscles hard, and without it, your muscles break down and what remains is fat. Having protein in your body means your metabolism is going to be faster, which means you'll lose weight faster. Of course, to hear some people talk about high-protein diets lately, you'd think it also cures baldness, makes you rich, and keeps you young forever.

The truth is, nobody stays happy on a high-protein diet. It's a no-win situation. After a while, it's a labor to actually move your jaw up and down. One recent study indicates a relationship between high protein intake and prostate cancer, and a Japanese study found a link between excess protein and diabetes. And since animal products that are high in protein are usually also high in saturated fats, they increase the risk for heart disease and stroke.

Just like there are good and bad carbs, there are good and bad proteins, too. Deli meats, hot dogs, sausages, and the like are known to increase the risk of type 2 diabetes, cardiovascular disease, and colon cancer. Poultry has saturated fats, too, but you can solve that problem by going skinless. Fish is typically less fatty than meat and is rich in omega-3 fatty acids, which are excellent for the heart. Of the vegetable proteins, beans are the absolute best. They have almost as much protein as meats, and since they're loaded with fiber, they suppress hunger longer. I love red beans, white beans, kidney beans, lima beans, and baked beans as long as there's no sugar or molasses in the preparation. My bean supreme, though, is the mighty lentil. Add a little olive oil and you can live on them. I'm also a big fan of protein shakes mixed with fresh fruit, especially in the mornings before a workout. The ones I drink contain about 40 grams of protein, and are low in sugar and fat.

CONFESSIONS OF A DELI GUY

In the early 1970s, I worked at the Dover Deli on Fifty-seventh Street and Lexington Avenue in Manhattan. I was the fish guy. In those long stretches between acting jobs, I'd spend my time cutting heads off sturgeon and slicing lox for ravenous Upper East Side New Yorkers. You can imagine what my aroma was like—never a problem getting a seat on the bus. But I was a real pro. They taught me how to slice lox so thin, you could read the *Daily News* through it.

I still love lox. The trick is to find lox that's not too salty, because salt will make you retain a lot of water, and being bloated to the point of resembling a small float is a definite drawback in the romance department. I tend to avoid full-fat cream cheese, though. Cream cheese will hurt you.

THE SKINNY ON FAT

You might have been surprised to read that my meals are 20 percent fat. That's actually a little low. Most experts recommend a daily fat intake between 20 and 30 percent of the total daily calories, though we can survive on as little as 10 percent.

With fats, there are good ones, bad ones, and frighteningly bad ones. Let's start with the monsters: trans fats, the unhealthiest of all. Trans fatty acids were first developed in the early 1900s as a cheap alternative to butter. By heating vegetable oil and bubbling hydrogen through it, chemists discovered a type of fat that could stay solid at room temperature. Soon, these solid fats, like shortening and hard margarine, became staples of every kitchen. These days, trans fats are the secret ingredients that keep packaged cookies, crackers, and chips "fresh" for so long. Microwave popcorn, margarines, instant noodle soups, and fried foods have some of the heaviest concentrations.

These mutant fats are among the real evils of modern eating. Trans fats weaken the heart and actually block the absorption of healthy fats. Researchers from the Harvard School of Public Health estimate that *hydrogenated fat is responsible for at least 30,000 premature heart disease deaths every year in the United States*. This is where reading labels can save your life. Beginning in 2006, the FDA will require food manufacturers to label the amounts of trans fats in their products. Until then, if you see words like "hydrogenated oil," "partially hydrogenated oil" or "modified oil"—or even just shortening—on a list of ingredients, turn and run.

As I'm sure you know, saturated fats, the ones from fattier animal products, are notoriously bad for your heart. I don't overdo it when it comes to red meat, but I eat enough to keep my iron levels up and because I like the taste.

Most of us don't eat nearly enough omega-3 fatty acids, one of two essential fatty acids. Omega-3s can reduce the risk for heart disease and cancer and are mostly found in fish and fish oil, green leafy foods, walnuts, and flaxseed. Flaxseed is so good for you but tastes so bad. But the good news is they finally figured out that if it didn't taste so disgusting, people would take it and, hence, live longer. Well, that day has come: it's now available cinnamon-flavored, so there's no excuse for not trying something that will help you live longer.

By far, my favorite fat is olive oil. Canola oil is exceptional also, and lately there's been some very positive buzz about the health benefits of macadamia nut oil. But you'll catch me drizzling olive oil over everything, breakfast, lunch, and dinner. It's loaded with monounsaturated fats, which enrich the body with vitamin E and antioxidants, and which is one of the reasons the Mediterraneans traditionally have such low incidence of coronary artery disease. It tastes great, too, especially some of the finer oils that are created with as much care as the best wines. If you want truly extraordinary oils, try Oli's extra virgin oil from Sicily, and anything from Capezzana or Castello di Cacchiano from Tuscany, La Cravenco or Huile d'Olives des Treilles from Provence, or McEvoy Ranch, a Tuscan-style oil maker from Northern California. And remember, unlike wine, the fresher the better.

GOING THE DISTANCE

If three out of four diets fail, is there any hope of losing weight and actually keeping it off? The National Weight Control Registry is a list of people who've lost at least 30 pounds and kept the weight off for one year or more. Here's what the world's happiest losers have in common:

1. Move: Every day. Take a half hour walk and combine it with things you should be doing anyway, like taking the stairs, playing with your kids, putting down the remote, and actually getting up to change the channel.

2. Eat Breakfast: A nutritious breakfast that's rich in fruits and fiber stops you from binge eating later in the day. For me, there's nothing better than hot Irish oatmeal with blueberries.

3. Weigh Yourself: The scale is the best lie detector. The registry's losers monitor their weight several times a week. That way, if you're gaining, you know you need to take action sooner to stay on track.

4. Read Labels: You'd be surprised how many calories, sugar, and fat some products have. Get used to reading ingredient lists and nutritional labels. It's your best defense against bringing fats and those bad carbs into your home.

5. Eat Smart: Smart weight losers generally limit the volume, the *amount,* of whatever they choose to eat. Portion size is three-quarters of the battle.

DAIRY PRODUCTS

Many people drop dairy products the second they decide to lose weight. That makes some sense, but I think people can lighten up in this area. Certainly, high-fat cheeses and milk products are notorious for their saturated fat content and for adding pounds. Cheese, cream, and other full-fat dairy products are best kept to a minimum. I love fresh raw butter, but it has twice as much saturated fat as meats, so use it sparingly.

On the other hand, at least one study suggests that calcium from *low-fat* dairy sources actually helps you lose weight, since extra calcium in a fat cell appears to burn more fat. I'm a big fan of 1 percent milk and low fat cheese. They're good for you and keep you looking robust. As you get older, your skin loses that layer of fat that gives you your healthy glow. A little extra milk fat now and then ensures you won't end up looking like a wizened old desert prospector. If you want to look younger and healthier, drink milk.

Then there's cottage cheese. I eat at least three pounds of Knudsen's pineapple cottage cheese a week, which is a terrific protein source and swimming with calcium.

JUICES

In the old days, everybody thought orange juice was the secret to staying healthy. It may help fight colds with its vitamin C and folic acid, but I'm not a big believer in it because too much orange juice is fattening and wreaks havoc on the stomach. It's like pouring tablespoon after tablespoon of sugar down your throat.

Far better are the juices, such as cranberry, tomato, prune, carrot, purple grape, and apple. Apple-nectar juice is especially high in vitamin A. In general, the cloudier the juice, the more nutritious it is. The juices you can see through are mostly water.

FOODS FOR DIGESTION

People hate to talk about it, but it's probably the single most important thing you can do for your body. Eliminating waste is the only way our

THE UNFRIENDLY SKIES

I'll never forget, I once flew back from Puerto Rico to New York and fell asleep just after they served me a dish of vanilla ice cream. When I woke up half an hour later, it was still sitting there, preserved in its own, well, preservatives. A little teardrop had melted off the top, but the main ball, the globe, the omnipotent vanilla muck at the center of the dish, was there for all to behold. It wasn't natural. I said to the head flight attendant, "Do you eat this?" And he said, "No. It's bad enough that we serve it."

And that was just dessert. The typical in-flight meal has more fat than a McDonald's burger and fries, according to a recent study by efit.com. Need more proof? How about this: I've never seen a flight attendant eat airplane food. Ever. What does that tell you?

bodies sweep harmful toxins out before they can do damage, and the best way to prevent such damage is to include plenty of natural fiber in your diet, or what they used to call "roughage."

During those intense stages when I was sticking to an all-protein regimen, one of the big drawbacks was feeling bound up from the lack of fiber. If you're on Atkins, South Beach, or any other high-protein diet, you probably know the feeling. Adding fiber is the way to go, literally. It reduces the risk of colon cancer, lowers cholesterol, and steadies your blood sugar level so you don't have that intense spike that leads to overeating.

Prune juice is a sensational fiber source, though many people reject it because it's identified with elderly constipated people. Get over that, because it's simply a perfect addition to breakfast! Nothing better. Whole oatmeal, kidney beans, barley, and chickpeas are great sources, too. My personal favorites are dates and figs. The natural fructose makes them delicious and they're phenomenal for the digestive system. When I travel, I insist that my family eat plenty of figs, preferably fresh ones, or prunes. And when we get to where we're going, particularly if it's after that long transatlantic or transpacific flight from Los Angeles, we all feel great. Flushing out all those toxins helps alleviate jet lag faster.

EATING TO YOUR HEART'S CONTENT—WEEKEND RETREAT!

And on the seventh day, you eat!

Nothing will work if it's too restrictive, nothing! Nature will rebel against anything that goes against it. Slashing calories, as a rule, goes against nature, which is why I allow myself one free day every week to eat anything I want. Anything. You can throw yourself into the world of ham-

WATER, WATER, EVERY DAY

Eight glasses. Ten glasses. A gallon. Lake Michigan.

Everybody has a different opinion about how much water we need every day to stay healthy and strong. I try not to worry about it, especially since there's little scientific evidence to confirm we need the standard eight glasses a day.

When I get up in the morning, I drink a tall glass first thing to replenish fluids and optimize the body's various systems. Your body will thank you. We get dehydrated at night. Then I'll have a glass at all my meals; sometimes I'll drink flavored water to liven things up. As you'll remember from sixth-grade science class, water accounts for roughly 60 percent of our total body weight, and even mild dehydration can tire you out, weaken your muscles, and kill your concentration.

Of course, the more you sweat, the more you need to drink. I start drinking water about 15 minutes before I get to the gym, drink while I'm working out and then drink to help my recovery for an hour or so after. It helps the joints stay loose and, if you're in weight-loss mode, it speeds the fat burning process. One tip: Drink cold water. The body needs to heat it, which requires more energy, which burns more calories.

burgers or pizza or French fries or ice cream or deep-fried chocolate candy bars. I usually start my break Saturday afternoon so I can go wild, and it still gives me the freedom to enjoy those waffles on Sunday morning and maybe a sub sandwich in front of a ball game on Sunday afternoon. By Sunday night, I'm actually craving a healthy change.

Believe it or not, the benefits are more than psychological. If you're restricting calories all the time, your body stores fat instead of burning it. That's why crash diets sometimes cause cellulite. The body begins hoarding fat, usually in all the wrong places. More important, I think a 24-hour furlough from the diet makes you feel human; it provides an outlet for our cravings and it gives us something to look forward to all week. Life's too short to never have Häagen-Daz's again.

This idea really came into play when I was on the strictest diet of my life for *Rocky III*. I had gotten down to around a much-too-thin 160 pounds, and I wanted my costar, Mr. T, to be around 205 so that we'd look somewhat in proportion during our fight scenes. That meant he had to lose about 30 pounds, which was a nightmare for a junk-food lover like him. Mr. T absolutely hated dieting. The only way I could convince him to do it was by giving him that one glorious day off each week. Still, we'd constantly find candy bar wrappers under the couch in his trailer.

But I'll never forget, we were shooting a grueling boxing scene and all week T's having tuna fish and vegetables or chicken and vegetables, and he's miserable. All he could talk about was the vanilla ice cream and cookies he was going to eat on Friday at five o'clock. Besides the role of Clubber Lang, that's all he was focused on. He must have planted the seed in my head, because I suddenly became as obsessed as he was. Vanilla ice cream, Friday, five o'clock. The whole set knew it. I think everybody in California knew.

Come Friday, we wrap the scene around five to five, and T and I literally sprint to our trailers. He gets to his first and I hear this bloodcurdling scream. Then I look in my freezer and basically have the same reaction. There it was, that horror of all ice cream horrors: not vanilla, not strawberry, not even chocolate, but a half-defrosted container of some green something, something like mint chip. It was a dark day for Rocky and Clubber. If I recall correctly, we attempted to flip the motor home over as a gesture of disappointment. Never mess with a man's ice cream; it could be fatal.

THE WAR AGAINST CRAVINGS

No matter how hard you try, no matter how long you've been "good," temptation is going to find you. It's not only you. Research shows that 97 percent of women and 68 percent of men regularly suffer from food cravings. Your three meals a day plus two snacks should keep your stomach happy but occasionally you simply won't be able to resist your cravings. Here's how I weather those storms:

★ DRINK WATER: Sometimes hunger is thirst in disguise. Drink a glass of water with fresh lemon and see if that does the trick.
★ WAIT: Cravings pass. Wait 15 minutes. Set a kitchen timer if you must. During that time, distract yourself with a phone call or a short walk.
★ CHEW SUGAR-FREE GUM: It just works sometimes.
★ EAT A BANANA: Okay, it's not pizza, but it will fill you up. If you're really desperate, put some honey on it.
★ SAVE IT FOR YOUR DAY OFF: Remember, you get a free day to eat anything you like.

HOLIDAY BITES

Holidays are supposed to be a break from reality. If you see some pie or stuffing you can't resist, I say go for it and know you'll pay the piper later. Promise yourself you'll stay on that treadmill an extra 15 minutes for two or three days and then you'll be even. It's very simple mathematics: whatever you put into your body, you can take away with the right combination of cardio and smart eating.

★ HAVE THREE BITES: I literally will order a whole pizza sometimes and just have three bites and walk away. Go outside anywhere for a couple of minutes. The hunger will pass quickly.

EATING YOUR WAY THROUGH THE DAY: THE MENUS

Here's what I eat during a typical week—meal by meal, craving by craving—to keep my body strong and my appetite under control. I think you'll find plenty of satisfying, easy-to-prepare meals that are really delicious. As you'll discover, it's a healthy eating plan but it's not a deprivation regimen. There are lots of carbs, fats, snacks, and, of course, the free day to enjoy whatever you want.

Remember: this is what I eat. But since we all have different tastes, I've also included a few suggestions for alternative meals. And don't be afraid to mix and match or make substitutions using my list of preferred foods on page 159. The purpose of these menus is simply to show you how to incorporate my recommendations for eating smart into your everyday life. *Buon appetito!*

Breakfast

Breakfast sets the tone for the whole day. If you skip it or run out the door with a cup of coffee and half a donut, I guarantee that by 10 o'clock your body will be clanging from hunger pangs. People think they can save calories by eating just one or two meals a day. That's not true. *Skipping one meal almost always leads to overeating at the next one.*

My breakfast rarely wavers. It's usually based around eggs or oatmeal. If there's no time for that, I'll have a protein shake, which is like eating two steaks with extra fiber and all the right nutrients. Here's what I eat, along with a few other suggestions for a week's worth of breakfast ideas:

Monday

1 cup oatmeal made from whole Irish oats, topped with blueberries and sliced banana

6 ounces pure tomato or prune juice

Tuesday

2 scrambled eggs in 1 tablespoon olive oil

1 slice whole grain toast with honey

6 ounces pure tomato, grapefruit, or pineapple juice

Wednesday

$1/2$ pound pineapple-flavored cottage cheese

Small fruit plate, including apple, banana, melon, grapes,
and figs or dates

Thursday

Three-egg spinach omelet

1 slice whole grain toast with honey

SEASON'S EATINGS

When I was a kid, the only seasonal ingredient I really thought about was canned cranberry sauce. Times have changed. Living in California, I'm blessed with some of the freshest fruits and vegetables in the world all year long. Fortunately, in recent years, farmers' markets and better grocery stores have been popping up around the country to put seasonal and organic produce within everyone's reach.

Paying attention to what's in season is my favorite way to keep my diet from getting stale. Many of these items aren't on my food list, because they're only available for a short time each year; that's what makes them so special. I really recommend seeking out farmers' markets in your area. That's where flavors are usually at their peak, and shopping at these markets is a way to support farming traditions that are being eroded by our urban society.

Probably the easiest way to know what's fresh is to look at what's cheapest in the market.

Friday

12- to 16-ounce protein shake blended with sliced banana and peach

Saturday

Whole wheat bagel, toasted and hollowed out, with smoked
  Scottish salmon
6 ounces pure tomato, grapefruit, or pineapple juice

Or I'll just eat the same thing every day. If you enjoy something, work around that food source until you get bored with it. The more repetitions, the easier it is to control!

SNACKS

It's essential that you never go hungry during the day, which is why I recommend having two snacks: one around 11:00 AM and one around 3:00 PM.

You should always feel like there's something inside providing comfort and energy. Some of these diet books drive me crazy with their tips for snacking: "Count out 11 cherry tomatoes" or "four ounces of low-fat Laughing Cow cheese pressed into celery." Try carrying that in your purse.

To me, a morning snack is an apple or a banana or a can of low-calorie protein pudding; if you have a few minutes and a blender available, make a protein shake. If you're feeling ambitious, you can make my cookies (see recipe, page 176) and snack on them throughout the day.

Some other snack options to enjoy in moderation include dates, unsalted cashews, peanuts, and pistachio nuts. Here are a few more options:

Protein pudding
Baked corn chips with black bean and corn salsa
A bowl of high-fiber cereal
2 teaspoons of peanut butter on whole grain bread
A health or protein bar

THE ROCKY COOKIE

When I was shooting the *Rocky* movies, I used small oatmeal cookies to keep my energy levels up. I was on a high-protein diet and needed the carbs, especially since I was exercising so intensely. Some days I'd down 30 or 40 of these. The cookies are about the size of a 50-cent piece and are made primarily of brown rice flour, whole wheat flour, and oats. In general, I recommend staying away from cookies and crackers, but these aren't bad if you need a little midday pick-me-up.

$1/_2$ cup whole wheat flour
$3/_8$ cup brown rice flour
$1/_4$ teaspoon baking soda
$1/_2$ tablespoon ground cinnamon
$1/_4$ teaspoon salt
$3/_8$ cup brown sugar
$3/_4$ cup Quaker Oats old-
　　fashioned rolled oats
$1/_2$ egg
$1/_4$ cup olive oil
2 tablespoons water
$1/_2$ tablespoon molasses

Preheat oven to 375 degrees. In a medium-size bowl, combine wheat flour and rice flour, baking soda, cinnamon, salt, brown sugar, and oats. Make an indentation in the center and add egg, olive oil, water, and molasses, and mix vigorously until the dough is moistened. Roll tablespoon-size balls and place 2 inches apart onto an ungreased cookie sheet. Bake 8 to 10 minutes or until done. Remove cookies from oven immediately and cool on wire rack. The cookies should be soft and slightly chewy.

THE MAGIC ELIXIR: APPLE CIDER VINEGAR

Apple cider vinegar is one of those fantastic elixirs that has been around forever. The ancient Egyptians used it to heal wounds and help cattle overcome fertility problems. Hippocrates, the father of medicine, found it worked as a natural antibiotic. Columbus carried barrels of it on his ships to prevent scurvy.

I've been using it for more than 30 years and I still swear by the stuff. Apple cider vinegar is produced by the fermentation of apples and contains cholesterol-reducing pectin as well as many minerals, including potassium, phosphorus, sodium, magnesium, calcium, sulfur, iron, fluorine, and silicon.

The first time I used it was around 1970. I contracted food poisoning and couldn't afford to go to the hospital. That's when I heard that apple cider vinegar has the ability to change the body's pH balance, which is so vital to good health. In its natural healthy state, the body is slightly alkaline. It must maintain that state to keep the systems in the body working together. But if the body is overly acidic, you are more likely to feel tired, get headaches, and develop digestive problems, urinary tract problems, colds, and flu. It's like two sides of a tennis court. One day you hit the ball onto the acid side and your immune system starts to run down. Cider gets the ball back on the good side of the court.

I thought it sounded crazy, but I took two teaspoons and the food poisoning was gone. Thirty years later, my wife and kids and my wife's sister and her children stopped to eat at a fast-food restaurant and everyone got deliriously sick. At my insistence, they picked up some apple cider vinegar. Each swilled a teaspoonful and they were back to their old selves an hour later.

Here's another benefit: Cider vinegar, besides curing or helping to cure what ails you, is a fantastic way to control diet and lose weight. Two capfuls in two ounces of apple juice can burn off more than 10 pounds a year.

LUNCH

Lunch is my core meal of the day, where I get most of the day's nutrients. There's still plenty of time to burn off calories, so I can handle bread, pasta, and grains. That said, I like to think ahead, so I don't overdo it at midday if there's a big dinner scheduled that night. I'll usually have a small bowl of pasta, some sort of whitefish in olive oil, grilled chicken, or a sandwich with the bread hollowed out of the crust. I'm a big fan of deli sandwiches and I know they are full of salt and saturated fats, so if I am to indulge, I save it for the weekend. Here are a few other lunch ideas to keep you going strong all week. Just use moderation. For dessert, try a can of protein pudding—it'll hold you for hours.

Monday

TUNA SANDWICH

1 can tuna salad, drained, with fat-free mayonnaise and fresh
  squeezed lemon, topped with dark greens and slice of tomato

1 slice whole grain bread, toasted

Apple, pear, or banana

Tuesday

RICE AND BEANS

1 cup brown rice with 1/2 cup black beans

1 ounce low-fat cheese, shredded

1 whole wheat tortilla

2 tablespoons fresh salsa

Wednesday

GRILLED CHICKEN BREAST

1 small skinless, boneless chicken breast, sliced and grilled with
  lemon and olive oil

Side of dark greens

1 slice whole grain bread

Thursday

SPINACH SALAD WITH CHICKEN

1 small grilled skinless, boneless chicken breast, sliced

1 pound fresh spinach

3/4 cup sliced mushroom

1/2 sliced tomato

1 tablespoon olive oil

1 hard-boiled egg, sliced

A handful of walnuts, chopped

Friday

PASTA IN OLIVE OIL AND GARLIC

1/4 cup olive oil

1/2 cup fresh Italian parsley, chopped

2 medium garlic cloves, finely chopped

1/4 cup chicken broth

7 ounces pasta of your choice

Saturday

TURKEY SANDWICH

1 whole wheat pita sandwich stuffed with 2 ounces fresh turkey
 breast, 1/2 sliced avocado, and dark green lettuce

1 cup lentil soup

1 apple or orange

DINNER

There's an old saying that goes, "Eat breakfast like a king, lunch like a prince, and dinner like a pauper." At the end of the day, food takes longer to digest, so it's smart to go easy on the calories. I try to cut back on starches, beans, and rich desserts at night. In other words, keep it simple. My dinners are almost always the same: I'll have grilled chicken or white-fish with some vegetables or else a small bowl of pasta in olive oil. And I always try to be done with dinner by eight o'clock if I'm going to bed around 11. The more you can stick to the same small groups of foods you enjoy, the easier it is to control weight. For example, I can eat steak or fillet of sole three times a week. So I alternate between the two, and I can therefore understand how to gain or lose weight by adjusting what I include as a side dish. But here are some other ideas for dining:

Monday

SALMON
Grilled salmon with lemon and fresh dill
1 cup steamed broccoli
$1/2$ cup brown rice

Tuesday

ROASTED CHICKEN
$1/4$ roasted chicken, skinless
$1/2$ cup baked sweet potato
1 cup steamed asparagus
1 sliced banana, sprinkled with brown sugar and cinnamon and
  broiled until sugar melts

Wednesday

FLOUNDER
Fillet of flounder
Dark green vegetables, steamed
Oven-baked carrots drizzled with honey
Small crusty whole grain baguette
Brown rice pudding

Thursday

PASTA AND MEATBALLS
6 ounces whole wheat pasta
5 small chicken meatballs with tomato sauce
Small green salad with olive oil and apple cider vinegar

"TO THE GOOD LIFE!"

I don't expect people to give up the happy juice with dinner. You've probably heard that red wine in moderation protects against certain cancers and heart disease, and can have a positive effect on cholesterol levels and blood pressure. You may need an extra couple of weeks at the end of the year to achieve your weight-loss goals, but at least you'll get there feeling like you've lived a little.

Crusty whole grain bread with olive oil and finely chopped garlic clove, toasted

Friday

KEBOBS

2 grilled shrimp and chicken kebobs with zucchini, peppers, and red onions, brushed with olive oil

Corn on the cob

2 Rocky Cookies (see page 176)

Saturday

CHOPS

2 medium lamb or pork chops

1/2 cup steamed sweet potatoes

Small green salad with olive oil and balsamic vinegar

Small crusty whole grain baguette

Small fruit salad

PARTING SHOT: SUPPLEMENTS

One last piece of advice: Use science. *Supplements give back what nature wants to take away.* In many health food stores, there are extraordinary weight-reducing supplements, weight-gaining supplements, brain-enhancing supplements, testosterone-boosting supplements, meal-replacing supplements. There are meal-replacement shakes that taste like milkshakes, which make an entire meal for lunch and even dinner. Want to make losing weight easier? Try protein pudding. Use supplements.

Believe me, I've been using supplements for 25 years and they've helped me achieve remarkable things with my body. I've also seen people transform miraculously before my eyes using them. Tommy Morrison in *Rocky V* came to me at about 205 pounds; we gave him megadoses of protein powder and such and he developed into a fantastic muscular specimen who eventually went on to defeat George Foreman for the heavyweight championship.

★

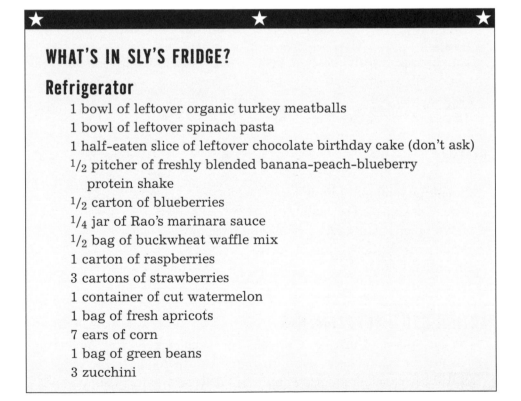

WHAT'S IN SLY'S FRIDGE?

Refrigerator

1 bowl of leftover organic turkey meatballs
1 bowl of leftover spinach pasta
1 half-eaten slice of leftover chocolate birthday cake (don't ask)
$1/2$ pitcher of freshly blended banana-peach-blueberry protein shake
$1/2$ carton of blueberries
$1/4$ jar of Rao's marinara sauce
$1/2$ bag of buckwheat waffle mix
1 carton of raspberries
3 cartons of strawberries
1 container of cut watermelon
1 bag of fresh apricots
7 ears of corn
1 bag of green beans
3 zucchini

1 yellow squash

1 bag of baby carrots

4 cucumbers

1 stalk of celery

3 heirloom tomatoes

2 heads of broccoli

1 carton of 1 percent milk

1 package of whole wheat tortillas

2 dozen large organic eggs

A bowl of grapes

1 small bottle of cinnamon flaxseed oil

1 jar of olives

1 jar of gourmet mustard

1 six-pack of protein pudding

3 containers of Yoplait Go-GURT yogurt (for the kids)

$1/2$ jar Danger Men Cooking Tough Guy Hot Sauce

$3/4$ bottle of Pepto Bismol

Freezer

Okay, you caught me—for the weekend:

1 quart Häagen-Daz's Cookies & Cream ice cream

1 quart Häagen-Daz's Chocolate ice cream

1 quart Häagen-Daz's Vanilla ice cream

1 quart Ben & Jerry's Chunky Monkey ice cream

1 box Tofutti Cuties

1 box of Dreyer's Whole Fruit Fruit Bars (strawberry, tangerine, raspberry)

2 boxes of Amy's Organic cheese pizza

7 packages of natural lean ground beef from Gelson's supermarket

2 packages of organic chicken from Gelson's

2 bags of vanilla bean coffee

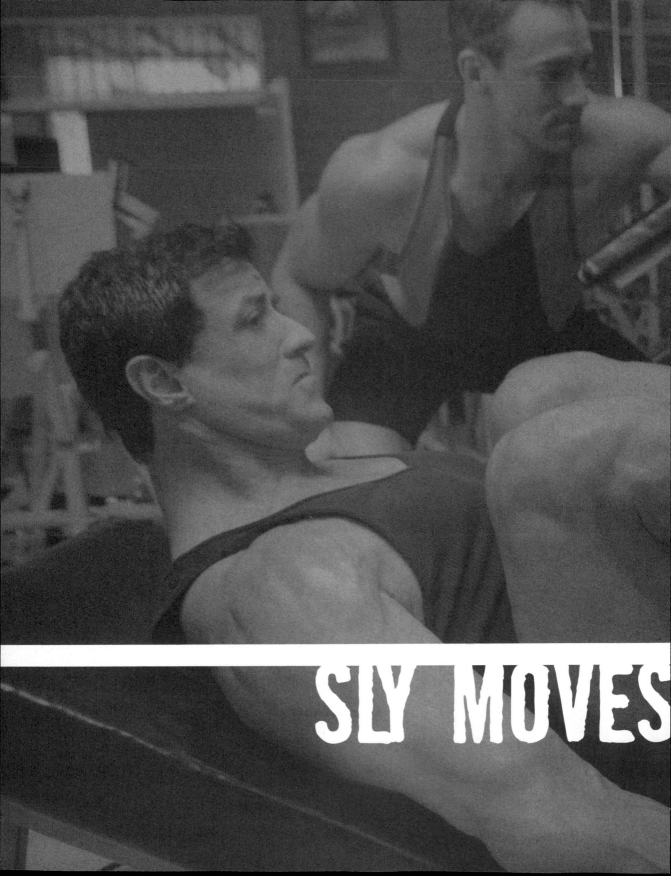

SLY MOVES

PART 4

IN ACTION

SLY'S TOP 10 TIPS FOR LIFE

10. Believe it! Truly, it can be done and it will.

9. Every day—every few hours—see your vision materializing.

8. Don't discuss your dreams. Pursue them!

7. If other people can steal your idea, most likely they will.

6. Don't be afraid of embarrassment while pursuing your goal. It's all part of being committed.

5. Being naïve in business and in understanding human nature is a recipe for disaster.

4. Study people's success stories hard. Study their failures even harder.

3. Enthusiasm is like a wonderful disease—keep spreading it until everyone's infected.

2. Only choose a goal that—if you had to—you'd gladly pursue for free. In order to achieve success, you've got to follow your passion.

1. Most important: If it's not broken, break it. That's how new discoveries are made. That's why everything that changes life is called a breakthrough.

You never know when you'll be called upon to rise to the occasion. For instance, when I was asked to carry the Olympic torch on its way to the 2004 games in Athens, I assumed I'd be just another anonymous runner in the longest relay on earth. But being the first torchbearer on U.S. soil turned out to be a bigger deal. That morning at Venice Beach, I was greeted by the mayor of Los Angeles, a Beach Boys–style surf band, and more than a thousand cheering onlookers with signs, noisemakers, and balloons.

Somebody had told me the run would be about 100 yards, but when I got there, it had stretched into a quarter-of-a-mile dash, mostly in heavy sand, and there was to be a parade of photojournalists jogging alongside me to capture the moment for the next morning's papers. *The last time I'd run along this beach was with Apollo Creed in 1983.* Bring on the pressure.

For two weeks, I'd been slowly increasing the slant on the treadmill to the point where I was practically running straight up a wall in the days before the relay. I'm not a born runner and I think it's totally overrated. When I was 16, we had to run a mile every day for the football team and I was always dead last. Finally, I got shin splints. But with this great honor of carrying the torch upon me, I knew I had a job to do and I wanted to make sure I was ready.

That's the way I see the programs for eating and exercise I've just laid out for you. They're all about being prepared. As you go through life,

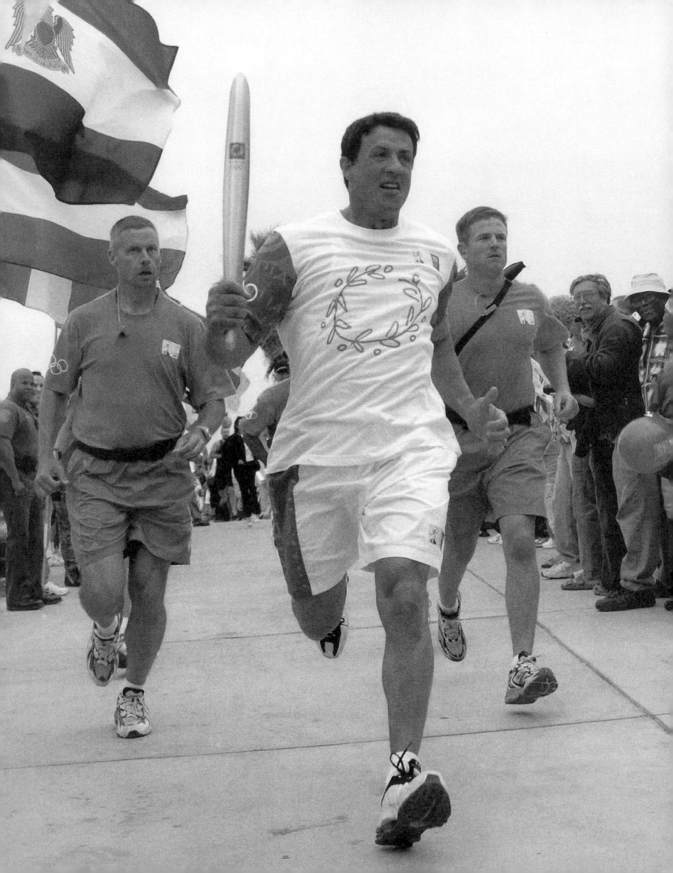

you're constantly faced with new situations, new challenges, new opportunities, and I can't think of one that doesn't benefit from having a strong and healthy body. You are like a good car. Your body is the chassis that carries you through all life's experiences, and whether you're 35 or 50 or 72, you want that chassis to function as well as it possibly can. Feed the engine properly and take it out for a spin on a regular basis. If you don't, just like a car, you will break down. Fast.

When you feel good physically, you're better equipped to take on the world. You are no longer a passive onlooker but are taking charge of the one thing you really have the power to change—*yourself.* You're activating your body so it can tackle any challenge that comes your way. When you feel good physically, you improve the way you feel emotionally, intellectually, sexually, and spiritually. You not only shape your own destiny, you inspire the people around you to live better, healthier lives.

In this section, I'd like to show you how I live by these words every single day. By seeing the ways I put my health and fitness principles into practice, maybe you'll discover strategies you can incorporate immediately into your life.

And, by the way, the torch run went great. I charged up the beach and through the crowd, feeling fantastic the whole time. I was so pumped, I ran straight past the person I was supposed to pass the torch to and kept going—can't take the ham out of the actor!

★

LEFT: First to run with the Olympic torch in the United States, Venice, California, 2004.

THREE DAYS WITH SLY
Day One

4:30 AM: Every molecule inside tells me to turn over and go back to sleep but I throw off the covers and get out of bed. Drinking a tall glass of water helps. It's my first order of business every morning. You just need it. You get dehydrated overnight and this is the best way to prime the pipes, to lubricate the chassis. Then I stretch. I do it every morning and I highly recommend it. Believe me, stretching at four-thirty in the morning is sheer torture. It really is. But there's no better way to tell your body it's time to start moving, to get the energy going. This morning I keep it gentle: I reach for the floor. It seems miles away. I hang there until my hamstring gives it up and finally my fingers touch the floor—and I'm off.

5:00 AM: I'm awake at this godforsaken hour to do some interviews with Philadelphia radio stations for my NBC reality show, *The Contender.* I don't get up this early for just anybody, but Philly's special. Long before I ran along the docks and up the steps in *Rocky*, Philadelphia was part of my soul. I spent my high school years there and the city helped make me who I am. I love its spirit. It's an underdog city, and that gives it a certain nobility.

When you do interviews, you try to stay focused on the project you're promoting, but I know these radio personalities, and, naturally, all roads lead back to *Rocky*, as if time has stood still. Or else they want to know about health, which is my second favorite subject. It's always the same thing: "Sylvester Stallone, you're almost sixty. How do you stay in shape? What is your secret?" I like to aggravate them. I tell them, "Nothing, really. I eat fried food. I stay in the sun. I smoke cigars. I drink toxic water."

6:45 AM: My greatest pleasure these days is spending time in the morning with my three girls—Sophia, Sistine, and Scarlett. I try to squeeze in as many physical activities with them as I can because we have so much fun. It's also so important to give kids an early start on physical fitness. The Game Boy generation, as I like to call it, has every reason in the world not to exercise, so we adults need to be good role models for our kids. Since the early 1970s, the percentage of American kids defined as overweight has more than doubled to about 15 percent, according to the Centers for Disease Control and Prevention. But research suggests that active parents who eat well and exercise often pass their habits on to their kids, just as sedentary parents do.

The big challenge with children is making sure they don't get bored. As soon as they've had their cereal, Sophia, my seven-year-old, and Sistine, my five-year-old, join me outside in the backyard and we swing golf clubs for 10 minutes. Next, we go inside and play billiards. It's important to build manual dexterity from a young age, and contrary to what most people think, billiards is a wonderful game for little kids. It does wonders for concentration and coordination. Sports of all kinds are so important for children and adolescents. I got into sports in high school—football, boxing, track—and it really gave me a focus. When my daughters get older, they'll be faced with a lot of temptation, a lot of peer pressure, and if they have activities that occupy them, they can release that energy instead of looking around for trouble.

8:00 AM: Since I'm not working out this morning, I don't require a great deal of caloric intake today. I have three eggs cooked in a wonderful Japanese oil that is polyunsaturated. I whip up a power protein drink with a banana thrown in. It tastes like a vanilla milkshake. For me, this is a perfect breakfast.

8:30 AM: We have a new puppy and I'm in training mode. If you want to get in good shape, get a puppy. Just chasing that monster around the backyard for 10 minutes works you out as well as any treadmill—especially this puppy. He's a Lousiana Catahoula Leopard dog, a breed that was used primarily to chase wild boar, so he'll fit into Hollywood perfectly.

9:00 AM: I read the morning newspapers from New York and Los Angeles and then start making various calls to see how different projects are going. I check in on my health supplements company, which is always a pleasant call because it's doing well. I'm putting out a magazine and I make some calls on that. I get a phone call about two TV series in development. Next, I check in with a director on a script I wrote many years ago that looks like it's coming back to life. It's a movie about the poet Edgar Allan Poe. He was an incredible genius who wrote some of the most haunting Gothic verse anybody ever put on the page. But the poor man died tragically at age 39. He was completely misunderstood and never really had the opportunity to show what he could do. I think a lot of people feel they don't get all the chances they deserve. I know I felt that way. He's a kindred spirit. That's why I'm always drawn to characters that have the odds stacked against them. They remind you you're not alone in the struggle.

11:30 AM: I rush to a *Contender* meeting with Jeffrey Katzenberg, the head of DreamWorks studio, and Mark Burnett, the creator of *Survivor* and *The Apprentice,* who's also overseeing *The Contender.* We're looking at hundreds of pictures and videos of boxers who'd like to be on the show and we've realized we have a monumental task ahead of us. There are so many compelling come-from-behind stories out there, so many overlooked winners, so many real-life Rockys. But it's hard to find the flowers through the weeds. Some of the guys have everything going for them yet they can't channel their energies the right way. Others are being sabotaged by misguided trainers or strong-armed by greedy managers. Others lack the vision to fulfill their dreams. It's incredible how many ways there are to hold yourself back in life. I've always used the obstacles around me as jumping-off points for new challenges.

1:45 PM: We break for lunch and once again I'm reminded how much bad food there is out there. Every day it's like walking through a minefield. You go to the office and somebody is offering you birthday cake. You need a quick bite and all you can find is fast food or fried food. You just have to be nimble, you have to watch your step and think on your feet. When the huge tray of fattening sandwiches comes around at our meeting, I decide to do a little creative reconstruction. I know how these things are done from my days behind the deli counter. There's always one sandwich that's all veggies, or one will have chicken with cheese on it. I'll take the sandwich and do a little counter-line surgery—take the bread and rip out the majority of the bulkiness to get rid of that calorie-rich white flour. You can still eat the delicious crust. Then I'll lose the avocado and cheese and put two or three sandwiches, worth of chicken on it, toss some extra lettuce on there, throw mustard on it, and you're there. Of course, everybody stares at me when I'm doing this, but guess what? Everybody's so competitive in Hollywood, they end up doing it, too.

5:30 PM: I'm back home and somebody calls offering me free courtside seats to tomorrow night's Lakers game. I say, "For sure."

7:00 PM: I meet George Foreman at Mr. Chow's restaurant. I'm running late because I want to produce a movie on George's amazing life and was meeting with a screenwriter who was pitching ideas for it. George, who's doing *The Contender* with me along with Sugar Ray, is one of my favorite people on the planet. Here's a man who thrives on change and life challenges. He's embraced one career after another, and each one is more successful than the last. He easily could have gone down a different path. Had he beaten Muhammad Ali in the "Rumble in the Jungle," God knows where he'd be today. But that loss taught him humility, it made him more human. Before that fight he was the ultimate villain. Afterward, he became the ultimate role model.

7:40 PM: George and I go back a long time. He and I have a lot of laughs and it's a fun night all around. Kirk Douglas and his wife come over to our table to say hello. So does Jackie Collins and Sidney Poitier's wife. A couple of rappers come to pay homage to George. Big, big George.

10:30 PM: I've been taking half an aspirin a day for 25 years, usually right before bed or when I wake up. I always do it. For years, researchers have known that a daily dose helps thin the blood and takes pressure off the organs and valves. It gives the body a break. We put such horrible things into our systems—food toxins, pollution, secondhand smoke, too many spirits—and aspirin helps counteract the damage.

Day Two

7:15 AM: Certain supplements really make a difference. In the mornings, I take blue-green algae pills, which sounds disgusting, especially with the word "kelp" all over the bottle, but they're incredibly good for you. Blue-green algae supplies all the necessary trace minerals that cause the body to work the way I believe it should work. It would require hours of foraging every day to get the same kinds of nutrients you get in two of these capsules. It's a giant antioxidant.

Nutrients that come from the sea have special qualities. I'm a big believer in using sea salt in my food, especially the sea salt that is derived from caves and hasn't been exposed to the elements.

10:45 AM: I work out three days a week for an hour to an hour and a half each time, usually on Mondays, Wednesdays, and Fridays. I go to Gunnar Peterson's private gym in Beverly Hills. It's a beautiful place to work out and a lot of celebrities go there, as well as some "normal" people. Gunnar's great. He's trained every athlete you can think of, including Pete Sampras and half the Lakers and dozens of the most famous actors in Hollywood.

I recommend people get to the gym 10 to 15 minutes before the time they intend to start working out. If you come in flustered, by the time you have your rhythm, half the workout's gone and you're not focused on it. I like to think of working out as a sporting event. You need time to get your game face. Plus, I like to make the rounds and say hi. You never know who's going to be there. This morning, it's Jennifer Lopez and Kim Basinger. Kim always looks fantastic. My wife thinks she's the most beautiful woman in the world, and part of her secret is that she's committed to working out on a very regular basis. As for Jennifer Lopez, she's also very serious about her fitness and she does a great job.

Today, for me, it's an upper-body workout. I work the chest, which means some seated rows, pulling the shoulder blades wide. Then I do some pull-downs. I do them unevenly, holding the bar in the center, and on the very edge, which creates an imbalance and in turn activates a new part of that muscle. Sometimes you can completely change an exercise by making one tiny adjustment. Even if you've done something a hundred times, you can bring new life to it with a minor modification.

Once the heart gets going, I down a bottle of protein amino drink, which really flushes the muscles and gives a little extra heft to them. I'm constantly drinking water, which some people forget to do.

12:30 PM: Lunch at home. Shrimp and snow peas, brown rice, lentils, sourdough bread. Half a liter of water. After a good workout, I feel okay eating a few more carbs.

2:15 PM: Back at *The Contender* office, I meet to discuss a few things with Mark Burnett. He comes from a military background and is in great shape. He was a paratrooper and he invented the Eco-Challenge. Mark has great confidence and it's paid off very well for him.

4:30 PM: Traffic, freeway-style. But I try to make the most of it. I have a thing about posture in the car. If I'm driving, I'll purposely put the seat upright to 90 degrees and try to drive with my head on the headrest, and it's so great for the neck and the spine. Or else I have my arms locked, which exercises the triceps, one of the most ignored muscles in the body. You'll notice that most people's biceps are in much better shape than their triceps. That's mainly because we're picking things up all day and pulling open doors. Triceps get built by pushing. The rest of the ride home for me is about steering-wheel push-ups.

5:45 PM: I've never become a slave to food or a serious connoisseur, mostly because I was never around good cooks growing up. Certain people I know live for food. With me, some days I'll eat amazing meals and other days I'll keep it incredibly simple. Tonight, I'll whip up some ribs. Basic beef in a light soy sauce. I stand in the kitchen with Jennifer and the kids, eating them out of a bowl. Why I bothered to buy a dining room table, I'll never know.

With our busy schedules and shuttling the kids around town, Jennifer and I sometimes don't get as much time to see each other as we'd like. But the time we do spend is wonderful. We joke a lot around the house. It's always mischievous with her. After dinner, she insists I have a piece of chocolate cake with her. How could I not give in to her?

8:30 PM: Staples Center, downtown Los Angeles. The Lakers are up by 10. Sitting at courtside is always a privilege and a pleasure, especially because they play the *Rocky* theme song. It's so funny for me when I realize these seven-foot giants were maybe a foot tall when the *Rocky* movies first came out.

Day Three

7:00 AM: I like to take ginkgo pills every day to help boost brainpower. We have to do anything to keep the pollutants out of our head, and ginkgo is one of the safest, time-tested natural ways to do it.

If you get into any kind of supplement regimen, I recommend keeping the pills at your bedside or in the bathroom. That way you remember them first thing in the morning. By the time you work your way to the kitchen, the phone calls start coming, the kids start screaming, and you're usually late for something. At least I am.

7:15 AM: I'm golfing today, so I can eat a little more. Breakfast is the time to do it, since you have the rest of the day to work it off. I eat half a whole wheat bagel with most of the bread part hollowed out. You need to be careful with bagels. They make them as big as tractor tires these days and they're loaded with calories. Go for whole wheat or whole grain. I like them toasted because that's easier on digestion. I also like raw butter rather than those fancy tofu/yogurt/buckwheat spreads. The fewer ingredients the better, as far as I'm concerned.

7:45 AM: I'm helping my daughters with their exercises. It's amazing how fast they progress. Two weeks ago they were complaining about doing 1 push up; now they breeze through 2 sets of 10 and brag about how no boy in class can come close.

9:00 AM: I'm signing some memorabilia for a charity auction. It's always so gratifying to me all these years later that people still connect with my characters. As a generation has grown older with Rocky, he now represents something new. When you're 25, Rocky is the guy who inspires you to take that first big chance, to "step up" even if people have doubted you since childhood. But at 40 or 50 and beyond, Rocky is still relevant. He sends a message to the world that says, "Don't ever count anyone out."

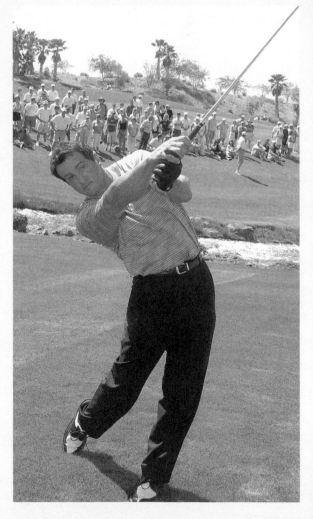

10:15 AM: I attempt to play golf once or twice a week. Golf is a terrific refuge for me, a green psychiatrist with 18 holes. It's also good exercise as long as you don't get lazy. I see these golf caddies who are 60 years old, and they're flying around the golf course carrying two bags on each shoulder. You want a good workout? Walk five miles through undulating fairways in 90-degree heat with a heavy bag of clubs on your back.

1:30 PM: I'm meeting with William Bratton, the chief of the LAPD, as part of my research for a film I may be directing for HBO about the deaths of rappers Biggie Smalls and Tupac Shakur, and the alleged police department corruption scandal that lurks beneath the story.

Heading out after the meeting, I take the stairs instead of the elevator like I always try to do.

3:30 PM: I am working on a *Rocky* musical, so I call Diane Warren, the Oscar-winning songwriter, to get her opinion on a few things. It's so amazing to me how this Rocky story just keeps giving and giving and giving.

7:45 PM: Dinner at Spago's in Beverly Hills with Jennifer and some of our good friends. Astronaut Buzz Aldrin and his wife are seated next to us, and I take a second to reflect on what an extraordinary figure this man is. The guy walked on the moon in 1969, and I'm thinking, I couldn't even get my car started in 1969.

11:15 PM: I'm really beat, but there's always one last item on the agenda. It helps me feel a little better in the morning. I end the day the way I start it, with a stretch. I have one of those inflatable exercise balls, which I recommend because it makes stretching easy and fun. I like how it helps open up the back when you sprawl backward on it. I do some back stretches and then throw in 25 quick sit-ups to shake off the day. Then I lie there and just breathe for four or five minutes. I'm thinking about all the things I've done during the day. I let go of the bad things, and I look ahead to what I have to do tomorrow. And there's always *plenty* to do tomorrow.

★

LEFT: At a celebrity golf tournament in Las Vegas, 2003.

GIVING STRESS A REST

Stress is nothing but a slow bullet to the heart. Study after study links prolonged anxiety to high blood pressure, heart disease, migraine headaches, allergies, asthma, digestive and skin disorders, obesity, sexual dysfunction, diabetes, depression, and more. The simple act of reading this is stressful. Some medical researchers estimate as much as 90 percent of illness and disease is partly stress-related.

Many people find balance through meditation, prayer, yoga, tai chi, massage, and old-fashioned talk therapy. Others get rid of stress by passing it on to others.

I've had as much stress as anybody over the years, and now I regard it like an unwanted houseguest that's a pain to evict. But eventually you throw it out, temporarily. Here are some ways I've managed to keep things under control.

1 START SLOW: If I begin the day in an agitated state, it's hard to get back on track. Rushing around to make an appointment or wolfing down breakfast to get out the door sets you up for a stressful day. If I know I've got to be somewhere early, I always set an earlier alarm to give myself a buffer. Even 10 extra minutes can make a huge difference.

2 CONSIDER THE SOURCE: People will always say nasty, negative, stress-inducing things like "If you haven't made it by the time you're 30, you're a failure"; "If you do/don't do this, you'll never amount to anything." Fine. But who's telling you this? Consider the source. Does that person have credibility? Do they have an agenda with you? Are they projecting something based on their own deep-seated shortcomings or anxieties? Could there be another side to the story? Don't be a fool by listening to a fool.

3 LAUGH IT OFF: A little humor gets people through the worst situations and the darkest days. I tend not to take things too seriously, especially as I've gotten older. It's the only way to survive. We're all here for what seems like two blinks of the eye. Then it's time to be replaced by the next generation. Life is over too fast to be bogged down constantly. Everyone gets down no matter who they are. It's natural. Deal with the problem quickly and move on. Postponing problems will lead to much bigger ones.

4 A LITTLE NAPPING GOES A LONG WAY: Often when we're feeling stress, it's because our bodies need a break. I'm not suggesting you sleep the afternoons away. That will make you even groggier. Ten or 15 minutes max is usually all you need to feel energized and to restore focus and a sense of peace. I recommend lying on the floor with your feet above your heart (rest your legs on a chair or couch), since that relieves the pressure on the joints, ankles, and feet and improves circulation. Just be sure the boss isn't looking.

5 SWEAT OFF THE STRESS: Exercise has always provided a tremendous release for me. There's no better stress buster than pumping the heart and getting the muscles moving. Numerous animal and human studies have shown that robust physical activity regulates levels of cortisol, norepinephrine, serotonin, and beta-endorphins, hormones that are essential for managing anxiety.

EYE OF THE TIGER: GETTING EVERYTHING YOU WANT

There are dozens of reasons why I *shouldn't* be where I am today. My birth was nearly botched. I grew up sickly. As an aspiring actor and writer, my drama teachers actively discouraged me, I had to beg to get auditions, and nobody would even touch my screenplays.

But even as I cleaned lion cages at the Bronx Zoo to cover the rent, I never lost sight of what I really wanted. With an income that never surpassed $1,600 a year, I waited seven full years to catch a break. Maybe it was the glow of youthful insanity, but I always felt I saw a faint light at the end of the tunnel. We take more risks when we're young, and rightly so, but I think doing things out of the ordinary as we mature is the best way to feel alive. Take chances.

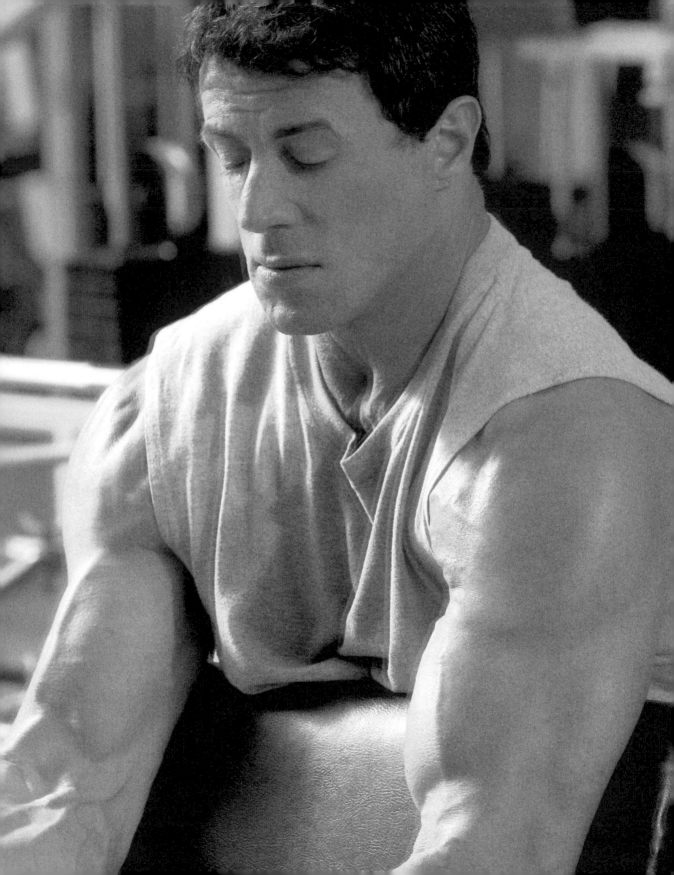

I see so many people out there who aren't living the way they want to live. They stay in cities and jobs and relationships and bodies they hate. They spend years envying other people's successes and relishing other people's failures. They're out of shape, out of energy, out of ideas about how to make necessary, positive changes.

Remember your dreams. We're nowhere without them. When I was very young, I started to visualize what I wanted to be and even what I wanted to look like. Those visions started to come into focus in my twenties. Even facing financial obscurity, I had an insane dream. The one thing that never cost any money was being able to visualize where I wanted to go in my life. And here's the amazing thing: seeing myself as a success tricked my mind into believing I really was a success. That's the sort of thinking that triggers winning streaks.

If you haven't asked yourself lately if you're living the way you want to live, now would be an excellent time. Is there still fire in your relationship? Are there still kingdoms left to conquer at work? Do you have the body you want and are you treating it the best way you know how?

Locked inside each of us is the person we want to be. Others might not recognize it yet, but I'm telling you, it's in there. The passion shouldn't die before we do. Even against ridiculous odds, what propels you forward and separates you from the rest? P.R.I.D.E., which stands for *perseverance, responsibility, integrity, determination, and excitement*. If you have these five elements in your life, you can accomplish almost anything.

Do a bit of soul-searching. Ask yourself some difficult questions: What do you really want? What kind of person do you want to be? And, when it comes to physical fitness, how do you want to look?

The clearer your goals and the more you refer to them, the more you visualize them, the easier it will be to turn those dreams into reality. And it's not necessary to share your aspirations with the people around you; some things should only be between you and yourself. I always found the longer I could keep a goal to myself, the more of a chance I had of achieving it. The more I talk about something, the less physical action I take.

LEFT: Sly today.

Throughout my career, I've used precise visualization to get what I want both professionally and especially physically. It started with Steve Reeves, who was the picture inside my head that drove me to the gym week after week.

If you're looking to make significant changes in your appearance, you need to know where you're going. Start a journal in a notebook or on your computer describing in simple terms what your health and fitness goals are. It's important to be realistic. It took me years to develop the physique I had for *Rocky* and *Rambo*. Don't pressure yourself to get six-pack abs if your belly looks more like a 10-gallon keg.

Write down your ultimate goals for your weight and waistline. I did this for years and still have these old yellow pages with descriptions of how large or small I hoped I would make each body part. I'd write the measurements for my chest, arms, legs, and calves. These were long-term goals. It helps to have a plan. Try building something without a solid blue-print. Some people will tell you it's possible to get the body you want in 12 weeks. Not true. But you will change for the better every day and one day soon you may glance up at your reflection while you're window shopping and you'll freeze. You'll study that reflection and smile. Why? Because you're going to like the new person you see staring out at you very much.

Once you know the big picture, block out a strategy. I find that tasks are much less daunting when I break them down into smaller pieces. That's definitely true of physical and nutritional goals. Here's what I recommend:

Come up with a list of 12 main goals and focus on achieving one a month. Month 1 might be about starting and sticking to a regular gym schedule. Month 2 could be losing 10 pounds by applying the eating strategies I've described in this book (you'll still be going to the gym, of course). Month 3 might be fitting into a favorite pair of old jeans by focusing on your lower body at the gym and continuing to eat smart. See how the goals start to meld into each other? At the end of the year, you will have worked your way to your goal without even noticing all the work you did. Well, that's not exactly true. You'll definitely notice the work you did because everybody will be noticing and commenting on how great you look.

Another helpful strategy is to use visual inspiration. Go through magazines and cut out pictures of people or even just headlines or words that make you feel motivated. I guarantee there's an image out there to inspire you. Personally, I like those before-and-after pictures of people who've gone from, say, 250 to 200 pounds. It just makes you think, "I can do that." You can even use yourself for this. At the start of each month, have someone take a "before" snapshot or Polaroid of you to track the changes you're making.

One other thing works really well for me, and that's accountability. Rest assured, I'm holding you accountable to your fitness goals, but I'll be honest, I don't have time to call each and every one of you to see how you're doing. My guess is, there's someone in your life you can count on to keep tabs on your progress, someone who can check in with you on a weekly or biweekly basis. That little bit of pressure and support is sometimes all you need to maintain your drive.

These aren't just great gym strategies, of course. They'll help you set and achieve goals in every aspect of your life, whether it's managing finances, changing careers, or improving your relationships. You'll benefit from the same techniques: setting clear priorities, breaking them down into smaller tasks, finding inspiration in images and words, and having someone who'll hold you accountable.

ADVICE TO MY DAUGHTERS ON LIVING WELL

Having young children in the house definitely keeps me honest. Kids see right through you and they haven't yet developed the internal censors adults have, so they're not afraid to tell it like it is. As they get older, I want my daughters to know what I didn't know at their ages about the way life really works. Perhaps I can spare them a few hard knocks. Here are some of my wishes for them:

1 NEVER BECOME FIXATED ON WEIGHT: It's so hard for young women in our culture to come of age without agonizing about calories, dieting, cellulite, and the rest of it. Men worry about their weight, too. But I want my girls to know deep inside that their value as human beings has nothing to do with the size of their waistline or how they look in a pair of jeans.

2 **DON'T TAKE OTHER PEOPLE'S OPINIONS TOO SERIOUSLY:** Most people give advice without really considering the other person. There's usually some personal agenda behind the advice, or the person has guilt, shame, or fear that's alleviated by telling other people how to behave. The only advice that counts for anything is the advice that comes from people who truly love you, or from your own heart.

3 **JEALOUSY IS A DISASTER:** Jealousy is a cancer on the soul. We waste so much time worrying about what other people are doing, what they're achieving, what kind of cars they're driving. It's absolutely useless, but for many people, the feelings never go away. I want my daughters to know that happiness can never come from the outside and will certainly never come from bitter rivalries or painful suspicion. I hope they will be able to free themselves from that burden—and it's an ongoing battle, because the truth is, jealousy is as natural as breathing. We have to tell ourselves to let it go. Once we stop fixating on other people's achievements we can tend to our own.

4 **THE WORD "NO" IS NONEXISTENT:** It's frightening to think where I'd be if I'd listened to all the rejections in my life. There's always a way to overcome a hurdle, to solve a problem, to defeat pessimism. It's never easy, but if life were easy, where would the motivation come from?

5 **ENJOY THE SPECTACLE:** I've come to see life as a giant passing parade. You never know what's going to float by or come screaming down the road. No matter what, it helps to enjoy the show. As my girls grow up, my wish for them is to appreciate the world around them, in all its pageantry and brilliance, and know that when the dark times come, those, too, shall pass.

RIGHT: Sophia and Jennifer
help Sly with his workout.

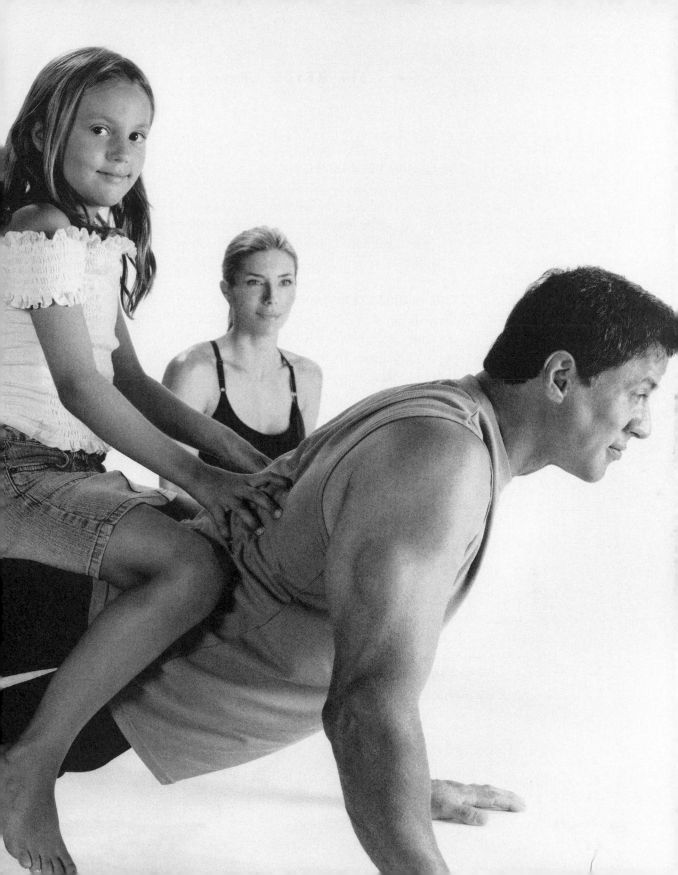

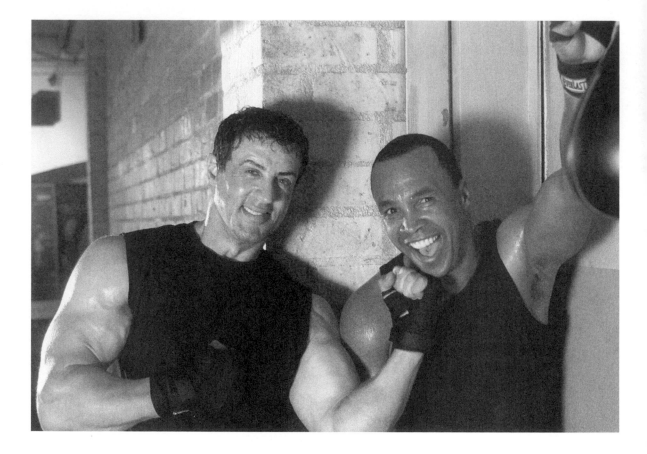

NOTES FROM THE CONTENDER

*T*he Contender was the closest thing I've seen to a real-life *Rocky* story, and I loved doing it. The reality show brought together a group of powerhouse underdogs with hard-luck tales you couldn't begin to make up. There was the East L.A. gangbanger and the hard-nosed Muslim from Detroit. One guy learned to box in prison. Another lived in his car for a year. Another surrendered to God and came out a Golden Glove champion.

ABOVE: Sly with Sugar Ray on
the set of The Contender.

We shot *The Contender* at a great big warehouse in Pasadena, California, and from day one, I discovered that reality TV is, well, a whole other reality. No scripts, no plots, no rules, no nothing. You're not playing a character. You're you and you're making a difference in people's lives. For the first time in my career, I was making an impact on the world around me instantaneously. Even scarier, there was no hiding, nobody to blame but myself if things went wrong.

I learned so many things from the experience, not the least of which was how undisciplined and uneducated even great athletes can be in the area of physical fitness. These boxers came in with such a mixture of good and bad habits. To compete on the show, each man needed to maintain a certain weight, and yet nearly half of them sabotaged themselves at one point or another.

One of the big shockers came when I went around their kitchen one day when they were out running. In the refrigerator I found a gallon and a half of ice cream, half eaten. Plus pizzas, frozen yogurt, tacos, and burritos. Further investigation uncovered Fig Newtons, jelly beans, cream cheese, bagels, Doritos, and bags and bags of pasta. I threw it all away and replaced the junk with what I considered perfect training foods: good proteins, healthy carbs, broccoli, sweet potatoes, cottage cheese, and olive oil.

Sure enough, six of the fighters came into my office with their game faces on and basically said, "We're grown men and you can't dictate to us what we eat." I said, "Look at me and look at you. I'm not even a fighter and I'm in better shape. And I'm twice your age." That quieted them down. For about 15 seconds. It wasn't long before they were gorging on all that stuff again, whipped cream and all.

So the moral of the story is whether you're a world-class athlete, a couch potato, or just an everyday person trying to do your best to look a little better, staying fit is an achievable goal—you just have to want it bad enough.

★

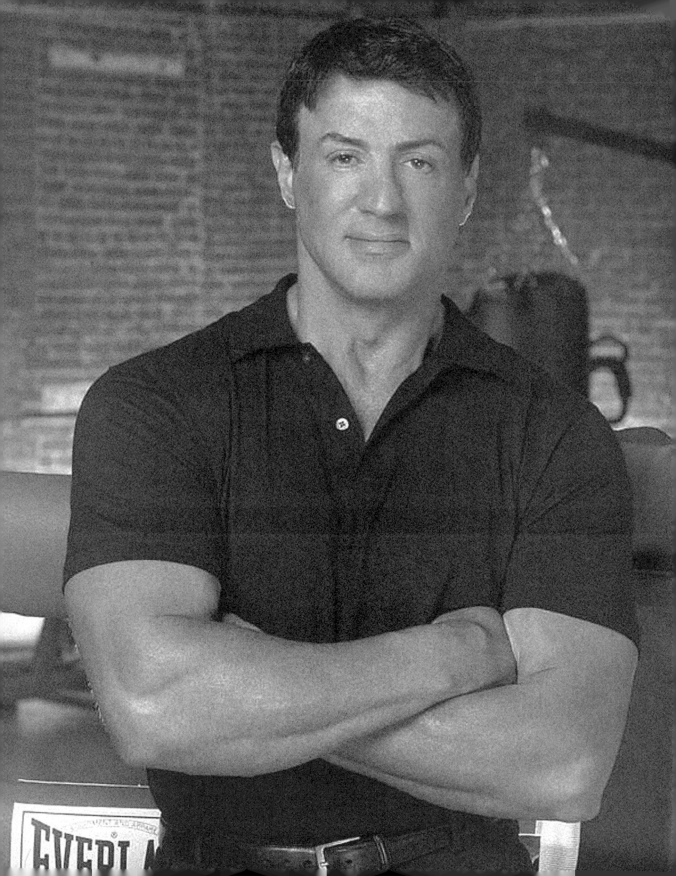

AFTERWORD:
GONNA FLY NOW

This isn't the end, of course, but just the beginning. You now have the blueprints to build a strong new foundation for your everyday life. With just a few changes, you can improve the way you eat, the way you shape your body, and, in turn, the way you look and feel.

The techniques and principles I've outlined grew out of years of experience, and they have definitely worked for me.

Years ago, as a young man, I wrote something that sounds overly sentimental today as I read it out loud, but it's the way I felt and still feel. Here it goes: "Once in one's life, for one mortal moment, one must make a grab for immortality, if not, one has not *lived,* only existed."

★

★ INDEX ★

Note: Page numbers in *italics* refer to photographs.